SURGEONS AT THE BAILEY

SURGEONS AT THE BAILEY

English Forensic Medicine to 1878

THOMAS ROGERS FORBES

YALE UNIVERSITY PRESS
New Haven and London

Published with assistance from the foundation
established in memory of Amasa Stone Mather, 1907.

Designed by Margaret E.B. Joyner
and set in Bembo type
by The Composing Room of Michigan.
Printed in the United States of America by
Halliday Lithograph, West Hanover, Massachusetts.

Library of Congress Cataloging in Publication Data

Forbes, Thomas Rogers, 1911–
Surgeons at the Bailey.

Bibliography: p. 235
Includes index.
1. Medical jurisprudence—England—History.
2. Forensic pathologists—England—History. 3. Surgeons
—England—History. I. Title. [DNLM: 1. Forensic
Medicine—History—England. 2. Jurisprudence—History—
England. W 611 FE5 F6s]
RA1022.G7F67 1985 614'.1'094212 85-8191
ISBN 0-300-03338-9

The paper in this book meets the guidelines for
permanence and durability of the Committee on
Production Guidelines for Book Longevity of the
Council on Library Resources.

10 9 8 7 6 5 4 3 2 1

To the memory of

John Hunter

and

Alfred Swaine Taylor

Contents

Illustrations

Tables

Foreword

THOMAS FORBES HAS ACHIEVED WITH REMARKABLE SUCCESS AN OBJECTIVE never yet accomplished, namely, an account of early English medical jurisprudence. The canvas for this is enormous. Let us look no further than the English records; they are compendious and, as the author discovered, reflect richly indeed both the personalities who gave innumerable notable trials their special qualities and the standards of expertise then extant in field and laboratory.

This is not just another review of the history of the period as reflected by the trial records of the famous Central Criminal Court. It is an instructive textbook of the art and expertise of the forensic specialist of the day in an area rich in English life, love, and licentiousness, yet grim in its medical ignorance.

We see surgeons and physicians seeking with a patent honesty of purpose to create a repute for forensic medicine and for the few scientific tests then operative and to achieve the acceptance of their evidence in the courtroom. The transparent honesty of the medical experts shines from the pages of the *Old Bailey Sessions Papers* in which the trials are recorded.

Forbes is plainly fascinated by such colorful if not always accurate experts as George Male, John Gordon Smith, Paris and Fonblanque, the Becks, Christison, and the great Alfred Swaine Taylor. Their influence on the development of forensic pathology is made evident.

This is a compendious work, reflecting the author's indefatigable interest. Immense pains have created an impressive accuracy of detail. The main body of material is culled from the trial records and arranged on a subject basis. All the questions that doctors and pathologists have to answer are set out here with a perceptive running commentary. It is fascinating to see the skills of bygone counsel parried by the learning—and sometimes wit—of the doctors. Forensic practice in court does not change.

The historian will be delighted with this new book, for it researches in great depth the English criminal trial records' wealth of material in an authoritative yet attractively modest way. Thomas Forbes' writing reflects his scholarly mind, and his pen runs easily. His excerpts from the trials will entrance the tyro and at the same time teach him much of practical court procedure. The expert will inevitably be delighted to read of his predecessors' trials in the witness box. It is always a joy to see colleagues—and their forebears—under pressure and to applaud their tactics and their skills under cross-examination.

Thomas Forbes has written a very scholarly book, researching early criminal trials in England with a perceptive skill that will ensure the success of this volume at all levels in both law and medicine. It cannot fail to attract both the professional historian and the armchair scholar.

London KEITH SIMPSON, C.B.E., M.D., LL.D.
June 1982

Acknowledgments

THIS PUBLICATION WAS SUPPORTED IN PART BY NIH GRANT LM 03266 from the National Library of Medicine.

Transcripts of Crown-copyright records in the Corporation of London Record Office and the Greater London Record Office (Middlesex Records) appear by permission of the Controller of H.M. Stationery Office.

The *Old Bailey Sessions Papers* were examined at the Guildhall Library in London. My best thanks go to Thomas Shaw, Keeper of Printed Books, and his staff for their friendly, skillful, and untiring assistance. Valuable help was also given by personnel of the Medical Library, Law Library, and Sterling Memorial Library of Yale University.

Keith Simpson read the entire manuscript; for this I shall always be grateful. Stanley W. Jackson and Franklin Robinson read chapters in their fields of expertise. My debt to them is also large. Albert E. J. Hollaender, Kenneth Keele, A. Keith Mant, David M. Paul, the late Ralph B. Pugh, and others generously answered questions and offered criticisms. Cinda D'Addio, June Connolly, and Selda Lippa graciously and accurately typed and retyped my pages. Most of all I thank my dear wife; without her support and encouragement this volume would never have been written.

SURGEONS AT THE BAILEY

Introduction

THIS BOOK SURVEYS ENGLISH FORENSIC MEDICINE AS IT WAS IN PAST centuries, before the days of fingerprinting, blood tests, and police photography.[1] In these pages we shall listen to medical men in the witness box at the Old Bailey, London's famed Central Criminal Court, as they tell of murder scenes inspected and bodies "opened" by the surgeon, and we shall consider evidence collected—and sometimes overlooked—that swayed judge and jury toward a verdict of guilty or not guilty. This account, less a history than a chronicle, covers the years from the Middle Ages to 1878, a long period during which forensic medicine made relatively few advances in England. This fact is the more surprising in that during the same time the science developed notably on the Continent.

But however much the English forensic expert lagged behind his French, Italian, and German counterparts, the juridical and social impact of his testimony was no less significant. Crimes involving violence to the person were commonplace, even though punishment was swift and severe for offenders who were caught. The English courts were busy. Time after time it was the expert witness, learned or

1. Forensic medicine may be defined as the presentation and application of medical information in a court of law. Strictly speaking, forensic medicine should be distinguished from the broader terms *legal medicine,* the application of medical knowledge to any aspect of law, and *medical jurisprudence,* which includes in addition the philosophy and science of law as applied to medicine (Black, 1968: pp. 777, 1133; Curran, 1975; Ficarra, 1977; pp. 3–4; J. G. Smith, 1821: p. 13). The term *forensic medicine* apparently first appeared in the title of Bohn's *Specimen Medicinae Forensis* (1690).

ignorant in forensic medicine, careful or perfunctory, concerned or casual, who in effect determined whether the accused perished on the gallows, were transported for forced labor in the colonies, or went free.

Research for this book was undertaken when, during study of London coroners' inquisitions and related papers from past centuries (Forbes, 1978), it became apparent that a comprehensive reconstruction of earlier forensic medicine in England was not available. Of course a good many popular and professional volumes reporting the investigation of notorious murder cases already stand on the shelves, including the accounts in the *State Trials* (Howell, 1816) and *Notable British Trials* (Hodge) series, but these books do not deal systematically with forensic medicine. There are also the technical works written in England and America beginning in 1816, when George Edward Male's *Epitome of Juridical or Forensic Medicine* appeared. But such volumes, particularly the earlier ones, were more concerned with principles than with specific cases, more with the theory of the science than with expert testimony from the witness stand. It was in the courtroom that the results of actual forensic medical investigation were revealed.

Rather like a good detective story, the testimony of the medical expert seizes the interest of the reader in several ways. The most obvious lure is the crime itself, that aberration of a human being who, in the grip of rage or jealousy, hate or fear, becomes the prey of explosive impulse, drunken confusion or, less often, of remorseless and calculating determination to kill. The crime is discovered, the law intervenes, the finding of witnesses and the gathering of evidence begins. Eventually the events are reconstructed for judge and jury as lay and expert witnesses give evidence.

In past centuries skilled, or supposedly skilled, court testimony came usually from a medical man, in most cases a surgeon. It was he who was concerned with the very center of the crime—the violence done to the victim, its methods and results. As we hear his unsparing account from the witness box, we are reminded of the paradox of forensic medical investigation: it is at once repellent and fascinating. Blood has spattered the wall; what do the position and shape of the drops tell the expert? What deadly secret, hidden in the victim's viscera, is disclosed by the autopsy surgeon's knife? The specialist's testimony may well determine for the jury whether the accused walks free into the sunlight or is led down a dark passage to prison and the rope.

Although documentation for this assumption is hard to come by, some portion of English forensic medicine before the end of the eighteenth century undoubtedly derived from the Continental school. News of important advances in Italy, Germany, France, and other countries crossed the Channel only, it seems, very slowly. Pathology, a sister science, did not even begin to bloom in Britain until the late 1700s, and Sir Robert Christison's *A Treatise on Poisons* (1829a), the first systematic compilation in English on the subject, appeared some decades later. For far too long the average expert medical witness in an English courtroom or inquest chamber was a busy surgeon, obliged to mount the witness box only a few times at most in his career and ill prepared for the experience. Unless he understood a foreign language, Continental lectures, books, and papers were beyond his reach. His medical education scarcely touched on the functions and duties of the expert witness, and the critical importance of useful medical testimony often escaped him—as it did the jurist and indeed the general public. When medical men did appear in court, it was to confirm the fact and more obvious circumstances of death. Very few of these witnesses understood how to search for evidence at the scene of the crime and at the autopsy table, how to record it accurately, and how to present it clearly and without equivocation. But as the eighteenth century drew to a close, concern grew within and without the medical profession that a doctor's training should include at least the fundamentals of forensic medicine (Medical, 1836, 1844). Books and papers began to appear on the subject, a few universities experimented with lectures on the new specialty, and legislation recognizing the importance of the forensic expert and facilitating his work was debated.

PUBLICATIONS

The first original publication in English to deal directly with what would come to be called forensic medicine was William Hunter's paper "On the Uncertainty of the Signs of Murder, in the Case of Bastard Children" (1783).[2] This landmark work, to be considered again in a later chapter, examined the difficulties in proving infanticide. A germinal wave of British publications had begun.

Five years later appeared Samuel Farr's textbook, *Elements of Medi-*

2. For a comprehensive list of early British and American works on forensic medicine, see appendix.

cal Jurisprudence (1788).[3] This first volume in English on the subject was, however, merely an abridged translation of the undistinguished *Elementa medicinae forensis* by a German, J. F. Faselius (1767). There followed brief works by William Dease in 1792 and O. W. Bartley in 1815, which contained little that was useful. Thomas Percival's *Medical Jurisprudence* (1794) was actually concerned almost entirely with medical ethics.

George E. Male's *An Epitome of Juridical or Forensic Medicine: For the Use of Medical Men, Coroners, and Barristers* (1816), was the first major, original book in English on the subject; solid, specific, and detailed, it included many references to the medical literature. About one-third of the work was devoted to poisons: their nature, remedies, tests for specific toxic substances, and the bodily changes observed at postmortem. The publication of a second edition in 1818 no doubt inspired the speedy appearance of other substantial volumes (David, 1973).

The first work in English on forensic medical aspects of mental illness seems to have been John Haslam's *Medical Jurisprudence of Insanity* (1817). The author explained in his preface, "The consideration, that in our own language, no work existed on the subject of Medical Jurisprudence, as it relates solely to Insanity, urged me to the present performance" (p. cclxxxiii). Although the work is a mixture of law and medicine, diffuse and often nonspecific, it did attempt to classify types of insanity. Thomas Cooper's *Tracts on Medical Jurisprudence* appeared in the same year. An American reprinting of the writings of Farr, Dease, Male, and Haslam, it also included shorter documents on forensic medicine, one of them a paper by Cooper himself on the detection of poison.

John Gordon Smith (1792–1833), the author of *The Principles of Forensic Medicine* (1821), graduated with highest honors in medicine from the University of Edinburgh in 1810. He became an army surgeon, served in that post until 1815, and then moved to London, where, however, his Scottish degree interfered with his practice. (In later years, as a political and medical reformer, Smith attempted—without success—to free the privilege to practice medicine from the barriers of national inequality.) His textbook was written during a four-year tenure as physician to the Duke of Sutherland. In 1825 and

3. After study at the University of Edinburgh, Samuel Farr (1741–95) earned an M.D. at Leyden. He practiced in Bristol and was elected a Fellow of the Royal Society.

1826 Smith lectured on medical jurisprudence, and in 1829 he was named the first Professor of Medical Jurisprudence at London University (Lee, 1909: J. G. Smith).

In September of that year Smith petitioned the Common Council of the City of London for appointment to the coronership of the City and Southwark, but he was not elected despite his obvious qualifications. A committee examining the office stated that "it will not be expedient for this court to confine the qualifications of the Candidates for the Office of Coroner, either to the Legal, Medical, or any particular profession, but that any Gentleman of experience, respectable Character, and liberal Education, is duly qualified to fill that office." Shortly thereafter, on 22 October Smith sought appointment as an associate of the coroner, pointing to "that assistance, which Medical Science only can impart." But the post went to another man, qualified neither in medicine nor law (Forbes, 1978: p. 9). Smith's *Forensic Medicine* complains that "in Great Britain it [medical jurisprudence] has been suffered to remain in relative obscurity until this day. . . . One thing is undeniable—that the testimony of medical practitioners on questions belonging to the department of Forensic Medicine has been conspicuous enough for discrepancy" (p. vi). The volume is systematic, lengthy, and detailed, "one of the best of the earlier books," in the opinion of Camps (1968: p. 11); it was followed in 1825 by *An Analysis of Medical Evidence* (1825). Tragically, Smith spent the last fifteen months of his short life in a debtor's prison, where he died on 16 September 1833.

Two other important books appeared in 1823, Paris and Fonblanque's *Medical Jurisprudence* and T. Romeyn Beck's *Elements of Medical Jurisprudence*. Paris was a physician, Fonblanque, a barrister. A good deal of the material in their three volumes and 1385 pages is not forensic medicine in the modern sense. Although it includes a useful exposition of the applications of forensic science, most of volume one consists of excerpts from trial records, the texts of laws and charters, and so on. Beck's book was the first significant American text in the field; J. B. Beck, a brother, was co-author of some of the later editions, several of which had British editors. The influence of these and other American works was felt on both sides of the Atlantic. James Webster's *An Essay on Medical Jurisprudence* (1824), his inaugural essay for the M.D. degree from the University of Pennsylvania, displays a commendable enthusiasm but little original material.

Sir Robert Christison (1797–1882) received his M.D. degree from the University of Edinburgh in 1819 and later returned there as Professor of Materia Medica after having worked as a house physician and having studied under John Abernethy, a London surgeon, and M. J. B. Orfila, the distinguished Paris toxicologist. Christison and a surgeon named Newbigging made the post-mortem examination of the woman for whose murder Burke and Hare were brought to trial in Edinburgh in 1828 (Christison, 1829a). His *Treatise on Poisons* (1829b) was soon recognized as a classic and went through several editions.

The publication of numerous volumes in the 1830s reflected an abrupt awakening of interest in forensic medicine and a recognition of the need to instruct British medical students and doctors in this neglected field. Isaac Ray's classic, *A Treatise on the Medical Jurisprudence of Insanity* (1838), appeared at this time, as did Charles Severn's *First Lines of the Practice of Midwifery* (1831), which had a section on feticide and infanticide. Towering among the forensic medical scientists was Alfred Swaine Taylor (1806–80) who, in the words of Simpson, "stood virtually unchallenged in his field for nearly forty years" (Taylor, 1869: p. 515). A pupil at St. Thomas's from 1823 to 1828, and then at Guy's Hospital, where he studied under the surgeons Joseph Henry Green and Astley Paston Cooper, the young Taylor particularly distinguished himself in anatomy—Beck's *Elements of Medical Jurisprudence* had stirred his interest in that field. He studied forensic medicine, anatomy, and physiology on the Continent and returned to London in 1831 as Lecturer on Medical Jurisprudence at Guy's. This post, established because of the commendable if belated decision by the Society of Apothecaries that candidates for diplomas must receive instruction in medical jurisprudence, provided the first official recognition of the field in England. Taylor continued at Guy's as Professor of Medical Jurisprudence until 1877, and also lectured in chemistry for most of the period.

His books, beginning with *Elements of Medical Jurisprudence* in 1836, grew encyclopedic in content and continued to appear throughout his life. *A Manual of Medical Jurisprudence,* first published in 1844, went through twelve editions, two of them after his death (1844a). *On Poisons in Relation to Medical Jurisprudence and Medicine* (1848), described as "the only major and truly authoritative work on the subject in English" (Myers, 1962), was published when the fourth and last (1845) edition of Christison on the same subject was becoming dated. *The Principles and Practice of Medical Jurisprudence* (1865), which was continued through many editions, was constantly revised on the basis of the author's enormous experience and wide reading of foreign books and journals. Taylor reportedly appeared as a witness in nearly all trials requiring a forensic medical expert during his professional life (Myers, 1962). Scientific articles also streamed from his pen: the *General Index to Guy's Hospital Reports* (General, 1894) alone names sixty-six.

Taylor's numerous publications were joined by other books in the field, although fewer titles were issued than in the 1830s, when a dozen first editions appeared (see appendix). Some went through several editions. The medical and legal professions had finally discerned the importance of forensic medicine.

UNIVERSITY LECTURES

The first university lectures on forensic medicine in Britain were given in 1789 at the University of Edinburgh, where Andrew Duncan, Sr., Professor of the Institutes of Medicine, delivered discourses on legal medicine and public health. Duncan had been much disturbed by the unsatisfactory and contradictory expert testimony in 1781 at the Donellan murder trial, held at the Assizes in Warwick, and determined to incorporate some forensic medicine into his innovative annual lectures on physiology. In 1791 he established a separate series of lectures for medical students on the new science, and four years later he published *Heads of Lectures on Medical Jurisprudence* (1795). The preface said, in part:

> Many questions come before Courts of Police where the opinion of medical practitioners is necessary either for the exculpation of innocence or the detection of guilt. . . .
>
> There is no branch of medical education from which a practitioner may not derive useful information on some points necessary for enabling him to deliver before Courts of Law, an opinion consistent with truth and with justice. (Littlejohn, 1928: p. 187)

In 1798 Duncan presented to the Patrons of the University of Edinburgh a memorial entitled "A Short View of the Extent and Importance of Medical Jurisprudence, Considered as a Branch of Education." A few years later the memorandum was recommended to the king's ministers by Henry Erskine, at that time Lord Advocate for Scotland (Duncan, 1807). It urged the importance of instruction in medical jurisprudence

> to every medical practitioner, who is liable to be called upon to illustrate any question comprehended under it before a court of justice. On his answers the fate of the accused person must often depend, both

> Judge and Jury regulating their decision by his opinion. On the other hand, while he is delivering his sentiments, his own reputation is before the bar of justice. The acuteness of the gentlemen of the law is universally acknowledged. . . . How cautious must, then, a medical practitioner be, when examined before such men, when it is their duty to expose his errors, and to magnify his uncertainties, till his evidence seem contradictory and absurd? (P. 244)

The document then discussed the functions of the medical police, concerned with the "application of the principles deduced from the different branches of medical knowledge, for the promotion, preservation, and restoration of general health" (p. 247). Most of the areas of responsibility enumerated were in the field of what is now considered public health.

Duncan's prolonged efforts ultimately met with success. In 1807 the British government created at the University of Edinburgh the first Professorship of Medical Jurisprudence in an English-speaking country; Andrew Duncan, Jr., was appointed to the post. A later incumbent (1822–77), Sir Robert Christison, carefully outlined his lectures in a *Syllabus* (1826). In 1833 the course in medical jurisprudence at Edinburgh was made compulsory. Distinguished successors of Christison in the chair included Thomas S. Traill, Sir Henry Littlejohn and his son, and Sir Sydney Smith.[4] Traill published his lectures in 1836.

John Gordon Smith apparently gave the first lectures on medical jurisprudence in England when he spoke in London in 1825 and 1826 at the Royal Institutions of Great Britain and also at the Mechanic's Institute.[5] In 1829 he became first incumbent of the Chair of Medical Jurisprudence at what is now University College. But instruction in the subject was not required for qualification by any of the licensing boards in London, and no students came to hear his lectures; after two years the unfortunate Smith resigned (Lee, 1909: 18, 491–92). A course in medical jurisprudence was thereupon introduced at the University of London by Anthony Thomson, the Professor of Materia Medica and Therapeutics. Thomson, a well-known physician who had helped to establish the Chelsea Dispensary and to edit the *Medical Repository*, gave his introductory lecture on 7 January 1831. In the same year Alfred Swaine Taylor was made Lecturer on Medical Juris-

4. Littlejohn, 1915: pp. 3–5; 1928: pp. 180–90; Camps, 1968: pp. 10–11.

5. I have not been able to confirm Sydney Smith's statement (1855) that "Dr. Michael Ryan began a course of lectures [in medical jurisprudence] in the Westminster School of Medicine about 1821." Ryan was not born until 1800.

prudence at Guy's Hospital, and George Burrows presented the *Introductory Lecture to a Course on Forensic Medicine, Delivered in the Anatomical Theatre of St. Bartholomew's Hospital*. Sir James Risdon Bennett, M.D., the first Lecturer in Medical Jurisprudence, Forensic Medicine, and Toxicology at Charing Cross Hospital Medical School, was appointed in 1838 (W. Hunter, 1914, p. 178; Charing Cross, 1838).

Organized medicine was at last coming awake. Burrows reported that "in compliance with the regulations for medical students, issued from the Court of Examiners [of the Society of Apothecaries], we have designated our course on Forensic Medicine" (1831: p. 6). In other words, some knowledge of the subject had become a prerequisite for medical licensure. According to Littlejohn, by 1831 the majority of the medical schools in Great Britain had lectureships in forensic medicine (1915: p. 4).

James Armour began lecturing on legal medicine in 1826 at the Portland School of Medicine in Glasgow, and was followed there in 1831 by J. M. Pagan. George Watt lectured in the same year and city at the Anderson College of Medicine. A professorship was created at the University of Glasgow by Queen Victoria in 1839.[6] Francis Ogston initiated lectures on medical jurisprudence at the University of Aberdeen in 1839 and from 1857 to 1883 held the professorship of that subject. He published *Lectures* in 1878 which dealt primarily with Scottish medicolegal procedure.

Burgeoning interest in the United States resulted in a series of addresses and books that were to find their way across the Atlantic to an increasingly receptive British readership. J. A. Stringham, who had received his M.D. degree from the University of Edinburgh in 1799, volunteered his services as a lecturer on medical jurisprudence in 1804 at the College of Physicians and Surgeons of New York and was awarded the chair in that field in 1813. The next year he published the syllabus of his lectures in *The American Medical and Philosophical Register* (1814).

The brilliant and versatile Benjamin Rush (1745–1813), like Stringham a medical graduate of Edinburgh, in 1811 found time to publish *Sixteen Introductory Lectures* on medicine. The last of these, "On the Study of Medical Jurisprudence," dealt almost entirely with medicolegal aspects of "those states of the mind which should incapacitate a man to dispose of his property, to bear witness in a court of justice, and exempt him from punishment for the commission of what

6. Glaister, 1928a: p. 418; 1928b: p. 202; Camps, 1968: p. 11.

are called crimes by the laws of our country" (pp. 365–66). Here were American roots of forensic psychiatry.

Charles Caldwell, "that belligerent Celt" (Garrison, p. 443), lectured in 1812–13 on legal medicine in Philadelphia at the University of Pennsylvania (Camps, 1968: p. 12). Some years later, in 1848, Dr. John Bell published a *Syllabus of a Course of Lectures on the Institutes of Medicine and Medical Jurisprudence, in Philadelphia Medical Institute* (Bell, 1848). When a chair of Midwifery and Medical Jurisprudence was established at Harvard in 1815, Walter Channing received the appointment, and in 1823 a professorship in the latter subject at Berkshire Medical Institution went to S. W. Williams (Camps, 1968: p. 13).

The brothers T. Romeyn Beck (1791–1855) and John B. Beck (1794–1851), whose works became well known in Britain, loomed large on the American forensic scene in the first half of the nineteenth century. John's early interest in forensic matters was already displayed in his medical thesis at the College of Physicians and Surgeons of Columbia University, *An Inaugural Dissertation on Infanticide* (1817). Eventually he became Professor of Medical Jurisprudence at that institution. T. R. Beck, the elder brother, had received his M.D. degree from Columbia University in 1811. Here he tells how as an American pioneer in his field he had to teach himself before he was ready to teach others:

> At an early period of my medical life, I became impressed with the necessity of greater attention to the science of MEDICAL JURISPRUDENCE, than is usually devoted to it by physicians. The writings in the English language on the subject, were at that time, confined to a small duodecimo volume, together with some detailed essays on particular points, and I soon ascertained that . . . I must resort to the study of continental authors. But my inland station, and the embarrassed state of the commerce of the country, seemed to present obstacles almost insurmountable to the acquisition of the systematic writers in question.
>
> During the late war [of 1812], however, a respected relative (The Rev. Dr. ROMEYN of New York,) while abroad, procured from different quarters the principal French authors on Medical Jurisprudence, and on his return, I had the pleasure of commencing its study with suitable materials. . . .
>
> My appointment in the WESTERN MEDICAL COLLEGE, rendered what had previously been a private study, a public duty; and I began to flatter myself that a publication on the subject might be found useful. The increasing attention to the science in Great Britain and this country, with the great facilities that of late years, have offered themselves,

> for obtaining scientific works from abroad, has encouraged me to prosecute my undertaking to its present termination. (Beck, T. R., 1823: pp. v–vi)

He acknowledged receiving "comparatively rare works from Germany and France," a tribute to his scholarship as well as his industry.[7]

Amos Dean, a lawyer but not a medical man, helped to organize the Albany Medical College in 1838; he became a member of its original faculty and served as professor of medical jurisprudence for over twenty years. Dean's *Manual of Medical Jurisprudence for the Use of His Class* appeared in 1840.

LEGISLATION AND ADMINISTRATION

Although the development of forensic medicine in England was assisted by the writing and teaching of medical practitioners, progress was at the same time seriously impeded by certain laws and administrative practices relating to the office and duties of coroners, to inquests, medical witnesses, and autopsies. The coronership, established in England in September 1194, had undergone considerable change over the centuries.[8] By the 1700s the office had reached a nadir of prestige and expertise, where it remained for many years.[9] An inadequately paid elected official, the coroner was not required to be legally or medically qualified. He usually received no additional compensation for conducting an inquest into a death unless a suspect had been seized who would be found guilty; only if conviction occurred did the coroner receive a portion of the prisoner's goods and chattels. So this official was seldom interested in accidental deaths or in murders by persons unknown. The system naturally encouraged corruption and neglect: many homicides were not investigated at all, or at best perfunctorily (Forbes, 1978a).

Centuries earlier, an act of 1487 (3 Hen. 7, c. 1) had authorized payment of a fee of 13*s*. 4*d*. to a coroner for each inquest held on a *slain*

7. Littlejohn, 1915; Walsh, 1919: 2, pp. 351–52, 357; Garrison, 1929: p. 769; Glaister, 1928a; Ackerknecht and Kozelka, 1950: pp. 1306–07; Camps, 1968a: p. 12; Nemec, 1976: p. 74.

8. For a review see Forbes, 1978a: pp. 5–7.

9. The history of the legislative and administrative basis for the investigation of violent and suspicious death is admirably discussed in chapter 4 of J. D. J. Havard's *The Detection of Secret Homicide* (1960). I shall attempt here little more than a summary of his observations and conclusions and those of Pilling, 1970; Mant, 1971, 1977; and Brodrick, 1971: pp. 112–14.

body; if death had resulted from accident or if the cause of homicidal death had been concealed, as in poisoning, the coroner had no incentive to investigate. In 1738 Parliament passed a law (12 Geo. 2, c. 29) allowing certain fees for services to be paid if the justices in quarter sessions approved. It took another act in 1751 (25 Geo. 2, c. 29) to specify that coroners could receive these fees: they were to be paid 20 *s.* for each inquest conducted and 9*d.* for each mile traveled. The 1751 act was intended both to encourage coroners to hold inquests whether violent deaths were felonious or not and to return some degree of prestige, usefulness, and integrity to the office. The statute further provided for a coroner's removal from his position upon conviction of "extortion, or wilful neglect of his duty, or misdemeanour in his office" (Brodrick, 1971: pp. 112–14).

Projected as a reform, the legislation failed. The coroners, quite properly, felt that *any* sudden and unexplained death should be investigated, but under the act of 1738 the justices could sanction fees only for an inquest "duly held." An inquest into a sudden death was usually considered unnecessary unless death was clearly due to violence; an inquest deemed unnecessary was ruled to have been not duly held, and payment to the coroner was refused. Such massive obstruction, which was to continue for a century, was, Havard states, "carried on in the face of incontrovertible evidence that they [the justices] were facilitating and inviting the concealment of murder" (1960: p. 38). These practices scarcely provided a climate conducive to the growth of forensic medicine.

A judicial decision in 1809 made matters worse. When the Kent justices withheld a coroner's fee on the grounds that the inquest had not been necessary, the High Court upheld the justices' absolute discretion in such matters. In addition, the travel allowance previously permitted to the coroners under the act of 1751, was reduced even though appreciable inflation had occurred in the interim; the restriction still existed in 1850.

In spite of the attitude of the courts, however, legislative attempts to reform the coronership continued. Two important acts were passed in 1836. One (6 & 7 Will. 4, c. 89) provided for the payment of fees for expert medical testimony at inquests and also for the performance of autopsies and chemical analyses related to deaths under investigation. For the first time the coroner was given explicit authority to order a medical man to perform these functions. The second piece of legislation, the Births and Deaths Registration Act (6 & 7 Will. 4, c. 86), established a national system of registrars intended to record every death in the country. But the law in fact applied only to burials conducted according to the practices of the Church of England and thus not to the interment of Dissenters, Roman Catholics, Jews, unbaptized children, and certain others. According to Havard, in the first year the act was in effect over 44,000 deaths were not registered (1960: p. 45).

The next year saw more trouble for the beleaguered coroner. A new act of Parliament (1 Vict., c. 68) authorized him to request reimbursement not only for fees he had paid to medical witnesses but also for the reasonable costs of an inquest. He was expected to disburse all expenses from his pocket at the conclusion of an inquest, then to seek compensation. But he could not be reimbursed until he had been examined under oath regarding his accounts by the justices of the peace at the quarter session. The coroner knew that these gentry, who took a dim view of inquests when the death was not obviously felonious—and of the use of medical witnesses in any event—might well refuse to compensate him for the fees he had paid. So he restricted his activities accordingly. A select committee appointed to look into the plight of the coroner failed to grasp the importance of expert medical evidence and published a report in 1840 accepting the position of the magistrates. Thus no reform was forthcoming, despite accumulating evidence of serious abuses, particularly in connection with deaths of children and deaths from poisoning. Burial clubs, in which parents enrolled their child for a relatively small fee and collected a substantial premium if it died, had become popular. The combination of a large family and grinding poverty was sometimes an overwhelming temptation to child homicide, which was easily accomplished, partly because of the widespread availability of laudanum and other opium preparations and the entirely inadequate control of the sale of poisons. Like other secret murderers, guilty parents faced little risk of detection.

William Farr (1807–83), the great Victorian statistician, leader in public health, and reformer, protested vigorously. Farr, medically educated, was compiler of abstracts in the office of the Registrar General from 1838 to 1879. During nearly all this time he composed pioneering studies, supported by evidence from his own statistical analyses of the causes of death in England and Wales; uncovered abuses in asylums and defects in the public health system; and pointed repeatedly to the dire results of interference with the proper functions of the coroner (Susser and Adelstein, 1975: pp. iii–vi). He was deeply interested in the accurate reporting of causes of death and had no patience with the inadequacies of the coroner system. In a letter appended to the *First Annual Report of the Registrar-General,* published in 1839, Farr, commenting on "the rude, cursory, *post mortem* examination," stated:

> it is not improbable that a certain number of cases of poisoning escape undetected by coroners and the juries, who can be expected to know little of the symptoms either of poisons or disease, and are very rarely assisted, as in other countries, in their decision by the information which a careful examination of the body and an analysis of the contents of the stomach would furnish. The result of this negligence is that little is known positively of the causes of sudden death; and the facility of procuring all the more intense poisons, as well as the prospect that the effects of poisoning *may be* confounded with natural causes, offers a strong temptation to the commission of that dreadful crime. Coroners' inquests are also held upon all prisoners who died in gaols, and the ordinary verdict is "Natural Death;" where it would appear that the inquest in gaols is at present very much a matter of form, although it was no doubt instituted to ascertain the real cause of death, whether it were a common disease, or gaol fever, or dysentery or violence. The causes of death registered as the result of a solemn, juridical investigation, are the most unintelligible in the register; as it is impossible to attach a specific idea to "Natural Death," to "Visitation of God," and to several other phrases in use in coroners' courts. (1839: p. 107)

Obstruction of the coroners' fees was again questioned in the courts in 1857, and once more the discretion of the justices was in large measure upheld. Finally, in 1860, the County Coroners Act (23 & 24 Vict., c. 85) placed the coroners on salary and made them largely independent of the justices. The annual numbers of inquests and of prosecutions for murder based on coroners' indictments increased conspicuously. In 1874, the medical man became legally obliged to fill out a death certificate if he had attended a patient in his or her last illness. Useful reforms in the coronership and in the registration of violent death were finally under way, although it would be a long time before the system achieved its present-day efficiency.

Another major impediment to the effective operation of the coroner's office was a widespread failure to realize that he ought to be trained legally or medically, preferably both. Instead, for centuries appointments were made on a political basis, and it was not until 1839 that Thomas Wakley was named the first medically qualified coroner for London. Member of Parliament for Finsbury and founder and first editor of the *Lancet,* Wakley was coroner for the County of Middlesex for twenty-three years. This vigorous and outspoken surgeon championed the reform of the coronership (Heddy, 1952; Thurston, 1969). The newspaper of the justices of the peace reacted predictably to Wakley's appointment: "It is not either in one case out of twenty that any medical skill is required, the cause of death being of itself sufficiently obvious" (Havard, 1960: p. 50).

We have seen how concern with forensic medicine grew in England in the first three-quarters of the nineteenth century and how the new science was promulgated in books and articles and in university lecture halls. Some knowledge of the subject, once the preoccupation of very few, eventually became a regular requirement for medical licensure. On the other hand, the proper functions of the coroner were seriously impeded by legal and administrative roadblocks which greatly retarded the development of forensic medical knowledge, the use of the expert medical witness at inquests, and, as a result, the courts' recognition of the importance of forensic medical testimony.

OLD BAILEY RECORDS

My reconstruction of the forensic medical scene in England was based in considerable part on testimony from the transcripts of actual criminal trials. Examination of the records of all English courts was of course impossible, but how about those of one major hall of justice? What better than the Old Bailey, London's renowned and venerable Central Criminal Court, site of criminal trials over more than three centuries for London, the County of Middlesex, and parts of Kent, Essex, and Surrey? So I came to the *Old Bailey Sessions Papers*.[10] Here, in the printed transcripts of hundreds of trials for homicide, assault, rape, and certain other offenses, beginning in 1684, were set down the learned testimony of surgeons, physicians, medical students, apothecaries, chemists, midwives, and empirics. Their testimony, "expert" in varying degrees, helped to send dozens of men and women—and some children—to prison or the gallows and to preserve the lives and liberty of others who in the eyes of the jury stood unjustly accused. Here indeed was forensic medicine in action.

The grim gray walls of the Old Bailey, London's famous criminal court, rise in the City on the street after which the massive building was named. A Sessions House erected there in 1539 was subsequently

10. Hereafter abbreviated as *OB*. Infrequently, silent correction of the punctuation in quoted passages has been necessary to make the meaning clear.

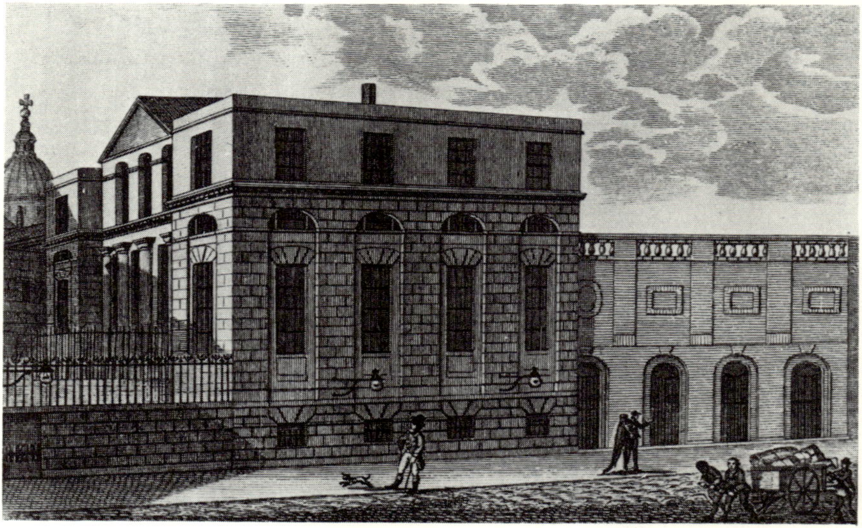

Session House, Old Bailey

enlarged, and in the eighteenth century the structure was officially described as Justice Hall. In November 1834 the Sessions House became known as the Central Criminal Court, established by an act of Parliament (4 & 5 Will. 4, c. 36) "for the more effective and uniform administration of justice in criminal cases in the metropolis and adjacent areas."[11] In *A Tale of Two Cities* Dickens told of the Old Bailey, "famous as a kind of deadly inn-yard, from which pale travellers set out continually, in carts and coaches, on a violent passage into the other world." (1906, bk. 2, chap. 2, p. 63).

Eight sessions of the court were held in a year that began on 1 December and ended on 30 November.[12] Although the court has always been busy, its official records other than the *Sessions Papers* were curiously limited, at least until late in the nineteenth century. Court rolls in longhand recorded the names of prisoners, the offenses with which they were charged, the relevant dates, the names of judges and jurymen, the verdicts, and the penalties for those found guilty, but *not* the testimony that had been heard.

By the latter part of the seventeenth century, however, enterpris-

11. Babington, 1971: pp. 24, 30, 189; Old Bailey, 1942; *Guide to the Contents,* 1963: *1,* 132; *OB,* Nov. 1834, title p.

12. The Lord Mayor of the City of London, wherein the Old Bailey stands, was, and is, elected for a term of twelve months.

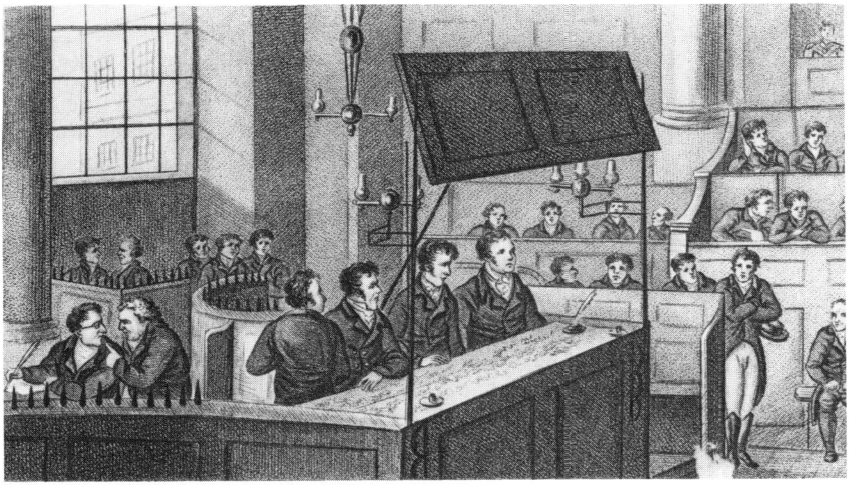

Interior of the Session House, Old Bailey

ing commercial printers had begun sending shorthand writers to court to take down the proceedings, apparently as a regular practice. From the shorthand notes were prepared abstracts, and later transcripts, edited to a greater or lesser degree (George, 1965; pp. 432–33; Walker, 1968: p. 57). Abridgment, it appears, was geared partly to the public interest in a case. Thus the excerpts of testimony selected in a routine trial of a pickpocket might total two or three paragraphs, whereas relatively little would be omitted from the account of a sensational murder trial. Editing involved deleting repetitions, irrelevancies, and other material judged not essential to the main facts of the case. No evidence has been found that the shorthand writers were legally trained, but by the early nineteenth century discussions of points of law were included or summarized. The judge's summing-up was almost always omitted. The transcripts were then assembled and published as pamphlets, of which there were one or more for each session. It is pretty clear that the whole process was a commercial venture with an eye to the interest of the public in general and also, in the nineteenth century, of the legal profession in particular.

The *Old Bailey Sessions Papers* are records of crime, of the prosecution and defense of the accused, and of verdict and sentence.[13] Be-

13. For an analysis of sentences handed down at the Old Bailey in 1729–1800 see Forbes, 1981a. Old Bailey trial transcripts reviewed for this book extended from 1684 to 1878.

tween the lines one can read much regarding poverty, social abuses, the criminal mind, attitudes of the public toward the wrongdoer, and changing ideas of justice. Together with the eighteenth-century *Accounts of the Ordinary, or Chaplain, of Newgate, which relate the Behaviour, Confession, and Dying Words of the Malefactors who were Executed at Tyburn,* published with the *Sessions Papers,* the records constitute a rich and fascinating store of information (George, 1965: pp. 432–33; Linebaugh, 1977: pp. 246–69).

Old Bailey Sessions Papers was and is a popular and convenient name for what were at first officially designated *The Proceedings at the Sessions of the Peace, Oyer and Terminer, for the City of London and County of Middlesex. . . .* In December 1774 the title was expanded to *The Proceedings on the King's Commissions of the Peace, Oyer and Terminer, and Gaol Delivery for the City of London; and also for the Gaol Delivery for the County of Middlesex, Held at Justice-Hall in the Old Bailey. . . .*[14]

The minutes of the Common Council of the City of London for 17 November 1775 recorded that "A MOTION was made and QUESTION put, That the whole Proceedings on the King's Commission of the Peace, Oyer and Terminer, and Gaol Delivery for the City of London, and also the Gaol Delivery for the County of Middlesex, held at Justice Hall in the Old Bailey, be regularly, as soon as possible after every Session, published by the Recorder, and authenticated with his Name: The same was resolved in the Affirmative" (*OB,* Dec. 1775, title p.). Accordingly, the title page for the ensuing *Sessions Papers* for a time carried the statement, "Revised and Published by John Glynn, Serjeant at Law, and Recorder of London." Later issues simply stated, "And Published by authority." The *Sessions Papers* continued to be on sale to the public.

The shorthand writers were anonymous until October, 1775, when "Taken in short hand by Joseph Gurney" appeared on the first page of a *Sessions Paper.* After 1775 the writers were regularly identified.[15] In the issue for December 1792 appears

THE OATH, TAKEN BY THE SHORT HAND WRITER, BEFORE THE LORD MAYOR.

You shall swear that you will, to the best of your Ability, truly take in Short Hand, the Proceedings on the King's Commission of Oyer and

14. "Gaol delivery" meant the emptying of a prison by bringing its inmates to trial.

15. Gurney was the author of *Brachygraphy, or Short-hand Made Easy* (1817). Charles Dickens for a time was a shorthand writer in the courts and the House of Commons.

> Terminer, and Gaol delivery of the City of London; and also the Gaol delivery for the County of Middlesex, and transmit the same fairly and correctly transcribed, to the Printer employed by the City of London.
>
> So help you God.
>
> Manoah Sibley.
>
> Sworn at the Mansion House, London, before JAMES SANDERSON, Mayor.
>
> (*OB,* Dec. 1792, p. 56)

Following Joseph Gurney, other early shorthand writers were E. Hodgson and the above-mentioned Sibley, "Professor of Short-Hand, No. 35, Goswell Street." The nineteenth-century writers included William Ramsey, Job Sibly, H. Buckler, James Drover Barnett, and Alexander Buckler. In at least one issue of the *Sessions Papers* the enterprising Hodgson took a full-page advertisement for his course in shorthand writing, his book on the subject, and back numbers of the *Papers* (*OB,* April 1790: p. 358).

The shorthand writers were not always merely passive observers. During a trial on 18 September 1854 a mentally disturbed man fired a pistol, fortunately not loaded correctly, at the head of a barrister appearing for the prosecution. James Barnett, busy as the shorthand

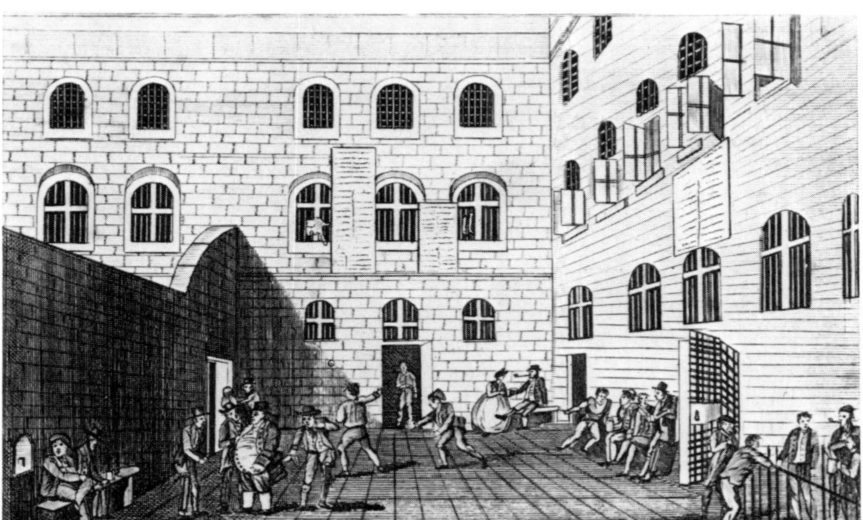

View of the Inside of Newgate

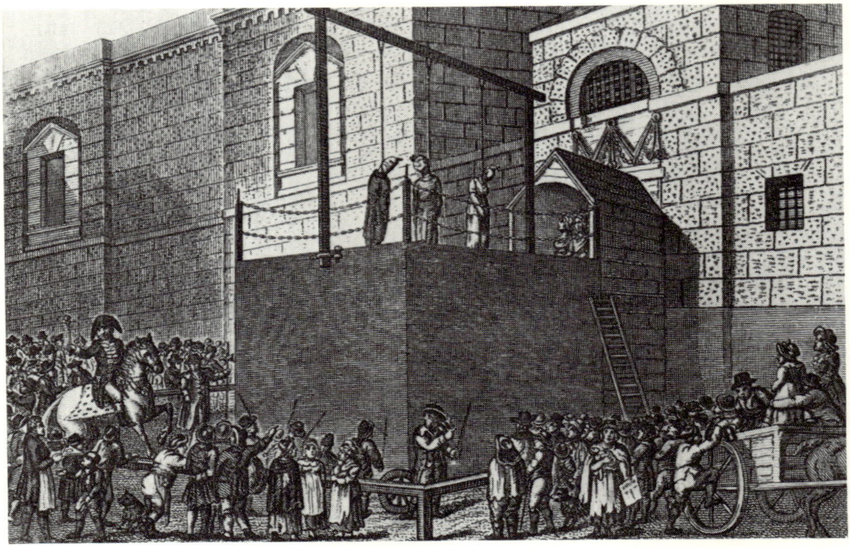

View of an Execution before the Debtor's Door of Newgate

writer in the court, crossed the room and disarmed the assailant, an act of some courage, as it turned out that the latter had a second pistol. The barrister escaped with a powder burn, and the bullet was found on the floor of the court (*OB,* Oct. 1854, pp. 1361–64).

In the seventeenth and eighteenth centuries crime was a formidable problem in London; offenses ranged from petty thievery to ingenious swindles to murder. The Old Bailey was kept busy, but many malefactors escaped arrest. Aged watchmen—the work was so badly paid that usually only the weak and elderly could be hired—were supposed to patrol the streets, but inertia, timidity, bribes, and threats of violence curbed their efforts. The novelist Henry Fielding and his blind half brother John, both magistrates, founded the Bow Street Runners late in the eighteenth century, officers who had some success in crime prevention and law enforcement. But the week-long Gordon riots in 1780 resulted in widespread loss of life, looting, and property destruction; Bow Street, the Bank of England, three prisons including Newgate, and many private buildings were burned. According to Paine, "At the commencement of the 19th century it was computed that there was one criminal for every 22 of the population" (1937: p. 158). In 1829 Sir Robert Peel organized the first police for metropolitan London, and subsequently the City of London Police, a separate body, came into being. Later action by Parliament extended a police system throughout Britain (Rumbelow, 1971: pp. 117–33). We shall listen to the testimony of watchmen, Bow Street Runners, and policemen in the pages of the *Sessions Papers*.

The file of the *Papers* at the Guildhall Library in London begins in 1684. There are many gaps until 1745, but the file is complete thereafter. In my search I scanned the available pages through 1878, finding over 2,600 cases involving some forensic medical testimony. Of these trials, 1,822 were for London homicides (table 1). The records of the most useful and interesting trials were photocopied for further analysis, and the cases reported in this book were selected from the latter.

Neither the *Old Bailey Sessions Papers* nor the present study include *civil* cases, even though medical opinion was required in certain common law actions, as in cases of alleged negligence resulting in injuries or in disputes as to the mental competence of an individual to marry,

Table 1. Old Bailey Homicide Trials, 1729–1878

	Homicide trials				
		With medical testimony			
	Without medical testimony	No autopsy report	Autopsy report	Total	% of trials with autopsy report
1729–38	44	21	45	110	40.9
1739–48[a]	30	13	14	57	24.6
1749–58	40	18	16	78	20.5
1759–68	47	22	15	84	17.9
1769–78	49	16	16	81	19.8
1779–88	28	20	16	64	25.0
1789–98	25	14	18	57	31.6
1799–08	30	11	14	55	39.3
1809–18	21	24	31	76	40.8
1819–28	33	32	48	113	42.5
1829–38	12	72	74	158	46.8
1839–48	4	78	119	201	59.2
1849–58	15	62	116	193	60.1
1859–68	13	81	140	234	59.8
1869–78	10	90	161	261	61.7
Total	401	574	843	1822	

[a]Incomplete; some *Sessions Papers* missing.

to enter into a contract, and so on (Havard, 1981: p. 813). Also deliberately omitted from this book are juries' decisions in trials where, for the sake of brevity, significant *non*medical testimony is excluded. Examples include the statements of a series of character witnesses or a discussion of a point of law by counsel and the judge. Often we need only a few medical particulars from a given case; to report the verdict might mislead the reader by implying that it was based on these details alone.

In table 1, "Homicides" includes all trials for "wilful murders" and for "killing and slaying," that is, manslaughter.[16] The latter term, incidentally, rarely appeared in the *Sessions Papers,* and then only after 1833. Because of the special legal and social status of infanticide (see chapter 6), trials for this offense are not included in table 1 but are summarized in table 4. The statistics in table 1 are for metropolitan London only. The actual number of homicides in a given year of course exceeded the number of trials for that offense. The number of trials was affected not only by population increases but by such factors as varying success in the detection of crimes and the vigor with which they were investigated and arrested persons were prosecuted. An extreme example of the latter variable is found in the Gordon riots of 1780, in which more than three hundred persons died (Rumbelow: p. 19). Yet there were only sixty-four trials for homicide in the decade of the riots, fewer than in the previous ten-year period (table 1). The rising number of homicide trials in the decade 1819–28 and thereafter, on the other hand, probably reflects primarily the increasing public concern with crime and disorder that finally stirred Parliament to enact remedial legislation.[17]

A conspicuous increase in the number of homicide trials at the Old Bailey is evident beginning in the decade after 1818 (table 1). The reasons for this increase are not entirely clear, but it coincides with the period during and after the establishment of the Metropolitan and City of London police forces. Also contributing to the increase in the number of homicide trials was London's growing population; the County of Middlesex, which formerly included London, had 831,181 inhabitants in 1801, 1,825,714 in 1841, and 3,779,728 in 1881 (Howarth, 1937:14, 355). No doubt other factors as well contributed to the numbers of arrests for manslaughter and murder in London.

16. Until 1752, New Year's Day in England was on 25 March, but the totals in the table are counted for decades beginning on 1 January.

17. As of 1978, London had about fifty murders annually (Simpson, 1978: p. 22).

CHANGES IN TRIAL PROCEDURE

English law was and is the product of a long evolution. Over the centuries there was slow modification of the conduct of trials, the rules of evidence, and the rights and obligations of counsel, the accused, the jurors, and judge. In future chapters we shall consider numerous Old Bailey trials. Since the reader may be confused by mention of certain courtroom practices that have now disappeared, we will briefly consider some of the changes affecting criminal trials.[18]

In the earlier Middle Ages, guilt was determined not by consideration of the evidence but by compurgation—in which twelve men of good standing in the neighborhood swore to the innocence of the accused—by ordeal, or by wager of battle. As these methods fell into disuse, it gradually became the jury which determined the verdict. The jurymen were local people who were expected to know the circumstances of the crime or to be able to discover them through inquiry. Thus instead of listening to evidence, as do their modern counterparts, the early jurors supplied it. They were expected to make a judgment as to guilt or innocence on the basis of their own information. The jurors were sworn to tell the truth and to reach a unanimous verdict; after all, it was said, there could not be two versions of the *veredictum,* that which is spoken truly. Even much later, when persons in addition to the jury were called into court to testify, the jury as a "body of witnesses" could still draw on its own private information. Not until about two centuries ago was the legitimate basis for a verdict limited to evidence presented in court.

The summoning of witnesses to testify before a jury seems to have begun around the start of the sixteenth century. The judge could exercise his discretion as to whether a witness should be permitted to give evidence. Holdsworth suggests that the court was more likely to call witnesses for the Crown than for the prisoner (1966: 5, 192). Until 1563 an accused person did not know who would appear to testify against him, and he could not arrange for witnesses who would testify for him. Only in that year was a law passed which compelled the attendance in court of witnesses, including those for the defense, and which invoked a penalty for perjury. Not until 1702 did Parliament

18. For the following discussion I have drawn on Stephen, 1883: pp. 416–17, 439, 441; 1890: p. 185; Hand, 1901; Odgers, 1901: pp. 216–17; Poland, 1901: pp. 50–51; Carter, 1910: p. 219; Jenks, 1912: pp. 350–51; Deans, 1921: pp. 142–43; Plucknett, 1956: pp. 136, 432, 435–437; Harding, 1966: pp. 127, 275. Holdsworth, 1966: 5, 192, 195; 9, 127, 131, 195, 214–17; 12, 507; Rembar, 1980: pp. 321, 387.

grant the right of defendants accused of felonies to have *sworn* witnesses testify in their defense.

Various categories of person were not permitted to give evidence in a criminal trial because they were, as the law said, "incompetent" to do so. Incompetent individuals included the accused and his or her spouse, although the former was allowed to make a statement at the very end of the trial. This restriction was indirectly modified by an act of 1848 (11 & 12 Vict., c. 42), whereby an individual was asked when arrested for a crime whether he wished to make a statement; the warning was added that anything he said would be written down and could be offered as evidence at his trial. Until 1842 anyone who had been convicted of a crime was also deemed incompetent to testify. Others who were barred from giving evidence were atheists, for whom the required oath was meaningless, and Moravians, Quakers, and Separatists, who refused to swear an oath. In 1861 the law was changed (24 & 25 Vict., c. 66), and these individuals were permitted to affirm instead of swearing.

By the end of the sixteenth century, information possessed by jurymen in a particular criminal case was no longer considered sufficient basis for a just verdict. Gradually, judges came to expect the "facts in issue" to be supplied instead by witnesses. As a result, juries were obliged to reach their verdicts on the basis of evidence, facts made available in court by witnesses or from documents, concrete objects, and so on. Certain rules evolved over the years as to what kinds of evidence could and could not be offered. A vast amount of descriptive and interpretative literature on this subject has accumulated; we need consider, fortunately, only a few points. One is that as the importance of testimony by witnesses became more evident, problems developed both as to the competence of a witness to testify and as to the degree of control a judge should exercise over what a witness had to say.

One point was firmly established as early as the seventeenth century—a witness could not be permitted to offer as testimony something that had been said by a person who was not in court. Such would be hearsay, second-hand evidence. By extension, the witness also was not allowed to give information derived from a document that was not produced in court. The exclusion of hearsay was "the most famous and characteristic of all the rules of the English law of evidence" (Holdsworth, 1966: 9, 214).

In homicide cases, however, an important exception to the hearsay rule was permitted. A statement made by a dying victim who was cognizant of the imminence of his death was admissible insofar as it related to the manner in which the fatal injuries were inflicted, or to other immediate causes of death, or to the person or persons believed to be responsible for that death. Such a statement was hearsay at the trial because its source was not available for cross-examination. For example, a man was brought into the London Hospital at about 11 A.M. on 28 June 1814 dying from injuries received when he was kicked and struck in the abdomen. His alleged assailant, Michael McGuire, was put on trial for manslaughter. The surgeon's beadle from the hospital was a witness:

> He was very ill indeed when brought in, and growing worse from the time he was brought in until he died.
>
> Q. Did he believe himself to be a dying man at the moment he was brought in?—*A*. He was told so by the magistrate when he took his deposition, and he believed himself to be a dying man. . . .
>
> Q. Now, while under the apprehension of his approaching death did he tell you anything?—*A*. He told me . . . there had been a quarrel with him and McGuire . . . he was dragged into an entry in the court, and kicked, and struck. I asked him particularly who did it; he said, McGuire.

The dying declaration was of forensic medical importance because it might be heard by an attending physician or surgeon who could be asked in court for his expert opinion as to whether the patient was indeed dying and knew it. Elwell adds, "The medical man should therefore note well the last words of the dying man, and the circumstances, and also his signs, for such signs, if *intelligible*, are also evidence" (1860: p. 318).

During the nineteenth century in particular, numerous legal reforms were introduced. Before then, whether investigation of a homicide should be continued beyond the inquest had really been up to the judge, and indeed some justices like Sir John Fielding made a conscientious effort to learn the details of a crime before the accused appeared in their courts. Other judges seemed not to trouble themselves. The establishment of London's Metropolitan Police in 1829 gradually relieved the court from the necessity of acting as investigator. For centuries, also, persons accused of treason or felony had been denied the help of counsel, a restriction justified "partly on the ground that the court was counsel for the prisoner . . . and partly on the ground that, it being for the prosecutor to prove his case so clearly that no defense to it was possible, no counsel was therefore needed" (Holdsworth, 1966: 5, 192). Not until 1837 was the law changed to permit counsel to assist prisoners accused of a felony (Plucknett, 1956: p. 435).

Sir John Jervis's act of 1848 (11 & 12 Vict., c. 42) made it mandatory that witnesses be examined while the accused was present, and also permitted him to examine them. In 1865 the Criminal Procedure Act (28 & 29 Vict., c. 18) introduced several further reforms. The prosecution, instead of occupying a privileged position in the courtroom, was reduced to a position of equality with the defense. Both sides were now allowed a second speech during the trial. If a witness produced by one side had at some time been found guilty of a felony, this fact could be revealed by the other side. Witnesses could be confronted with, and even examined on, their pretrial statements. The Crown could not attempt to discredit a prosecution witness if he were discovered to be favorable to the prisoner. In 1867 it became possible for the accused, equally with the prosecution, to call a witness for testimony *before* the trial, and such a witness could be obliged to attend the trial.

THE EXPERT WITNESS

Of all those who may testify, the key figure from the standpoint of forensic medicine is of course the expert witness. In the eyes of the law he occupies a special position, for he possesses knowledge and skill not shared by all. Indeed, when the medical man comes to the stand counsel may require him to establish his expertise by describing his special training and experience. The expert witness is also unique because he may give evidence in the form of *opinion* as well as of fact. (Hand [1901] points out that from the metaphysical standpoint it is difficult to distinguish between fact and opinion, since the acceptance of a fact is based on the opinion that it is a fact.)

The distinction between evidentiary fact and evidentiary opinion can be viewed historically. Consider the trial for witchcraft held at Bury St. Edmunds in March 1665. Some children, it was alleged, suddenly began to suffer from fits and vomited forty or more crooked pins and "a two-penny nail with a very broad head." Obviously, said parents and friends, the children were the victims of sorcery. The women held responsible were brought to trial. Among those in the courtroom was the learned Dr. Brown of Norwich. Questioned as an expert witness, he remarked first that Denmark had recently had an outbreak of the same kind of bewitchment, and then went on to explain that the children's fits and other afflictions had a scientific explanation. They were caused by the devil who "did work upon the bodies of men and women, upon a natural foundation, (that is) to stir up and excite such humours super-abounding in their bodies to a great excess." The swooning fits were "natural . . . but only heightened to a great excess by the subtilty of the devil" (Howell, 1816: 6, cols. 687–97). Three hundred years later Dr. Brown's scientific facts are reduced in our eyes to his opinions. But it is only fair to add that in some areas of forensic medicine, notably in the insanity defense, the struggle to separate fact from opinion still goes on.

Two of the methods for eliciting expert information are, as Hand points out, very old and have since been replaced by the testimony of the expert witness to the jury. In one method the judge simply selected jurymen with the requisite special knowledge, while in the other he sought in advance of the trial and for his own guidance the opinions of specially qualified individuals. The great Henry de Bracton, a thirteenth-century ecclesiastic and judge, used the latter method. In his compendious treatise on English law Bracton specified the form of what came to be called a writ *de ventre inspiciendo* ("concerning the examination of the belly" [*De legibus et consuetudinibus Angliae,* 6k. 2, fol. 69; quoted by Thorne, 1968: pp. 201–02]). Such an examination might be required by the court in the case of a birth suppositiously or fraudulently pretended in support of claims to inherit. The inspection was to be made "a discretis mulieribus, et tractari per ubera et per ventrem, ad inquirendam veritatem" ("by responsible matrons and by palpating the breasts and abdomen to determine the truth"). Of course the responsible matrons were not medical men, who would not have been permitted in any case to examine a woman in such manner, but by definition the matrons would probably have experienced pregnancy themselves and might even in some cases be midwives—as close as the court could come to experts under the circumstances. Utilization of the medical witness seems to have been well established by the sixteenth century (Holdsworth, 1966: 5, 419).

When the validity of expert medical testimony was challenged, a number of secondary problems were engendered. Counsel would sometimes attack the professional competence of the witness. The renowned William Hunter (1718–83) did not hesitate to acknowledge that many members "of our profession are not so conversant with science as the world may think." Some of these individuals, he remarked, could not resist the temptation to deliver "a quick and decided opinion." Support for Hunter's contention is not lacking in the pages of trial records. A conflict in medical testimony placed the burden of choice between experts on the shoulders of the jury and the judge. Listen, for example, to Mr. Baron Alderson, presiding at a trial in 1849:

> What are "the facts proved?" Is Dr. Sutherland [the witness] to be the Judge, or the Jury and I? It implies that the facts are proved; there are no facts proved at present. . . . The way to examine a scientific witness is to put general questions to him, such as "What are the symptoms of insanity?" "In what way do you judge such a symptom to be one of insanity or the reverse?" and the Jury will apply his hypothetic answer to the facts before them; if it agrees with the facts, they will apply the opinion; if not, it goes for nothing. (*OB,* Nov. 1849: pp. 39–50)

Hand observes that if the jury believed an expert, he took the jury's place; that is, the verdict was then, in effect, in the hands of the expert (1901).

In 1851 Storer, lecturing on medical jurisprudence, emphasized that the expert witness must "state the facts, at all events, as he knows them"; he must be truthful (1851: p. 10). Quite so. But one has the impression that contradictory expert testimony usually had its origin not in dishonesty but in honest difference of opinion. In either case the expert, having become "a hired champion of one side . . . is the subject of examination and cross-examination and of contradiction by other experts" (Hand, 1901).

Such disagreement naturally was fuel for the hot fires of the adversary process, expertly tended by opposing counsel, as in the following effort to shake the credibility of a midwife giving testimony in the case of a young woman charged with infanticide:

> *Cross-examined by Mr. Knapp. Q.* Do you mean to swear positively that the child you examined was born alive?—*A.* No, I do not, but to the best of my knowledge it was.
>
> *Q.* Do you mean to be understood, that you have always said you believed the child was born alive?—*A.* Yes, I do, it was.
>
> *Q.* Have you always said so, clear as you do now?—*A.* I don't know anything to the contrary.
>
> *Q.* Upon your oath, did you not before the Magistrate [at the preliminary hearing] entertain a doubt whether the child was born alive or not?—*A.* No.
>
> *Q.* You never entertained any doubt?—No. . . .
>
> *Court. Q.* I want to know what it is you do mean; when I read your deposition before the Alderman, I was led to suppose that it amounted to your idea, and to the best of your opinion; I understand you will not now swear it as a positive fact?—*A.* I cannot swear it as a positive fact, though I believe it. (*OB,* Sept. 1802: pp. 460–62)

The expert's scientific terms when not explained in simple language confounded the layman. Consider the bewilderment of shopkeepers, clerks, and journeymen in the jury box confronted with *mesenteric glands, trepan, pleura, fomentation,* and *monomania.* Experienced medical witnesses often seemed to be aware of this problem and made an effort to explain technical matters.

Sometimes the judge took it on himself to assist or even direct the jury regarding expert testimony. When he was unwilling or unable to do so, the jurymen had to struggle on as best they could. In a 1786 murder trial an apothecary was being questioned:

> Have you a real doubt in your mind what that fever was caused by?—[Apothecary.] There is a probability that it might be occasioned from intoxication, from passion, from anger; or it might be from the falls he received; it is very doubtful to me.
>
> *Mr. Justice Gould.* I take the case to be that the cause of death must be proved and drawn from a variety of circumstances; the Court are to form their judgement from the evidence they have heard, and if they are of opinion that the death arose from the ill usage given, by that prisoner at the bar, certainly the fact is proved; the fact is to be proved from the result of all the evidence, duly weighed and adjudged by the Jury, the Jury are to judge for themselves; suppose a surgeon was to say, where it was manifestly clear that the injury was the occasion of the death, that he was of opinion that it was not; is that to blind the Jury? they are not be be hood-winked or blinded; though not persons of professional skill, they are endued with common sense. . . . Surgeons are called only to assist your judgment, they are not the people to determine this or any other case. (*OB,* Aug. 1786: pp. 1130–39)

In a later trial the judge again left the unfortunate jury to decide between experts.

> Gentlemen [of the Jury], thus far I ought to state . . . that from the result of the opinions of these medical gentlemen, it seems to be uncertain whether the death be attributable to those means which the [coroner's] inquisition ascribes [i.e., murder], or whether it might not have arisen from intoxication. . . . it will be for you to draw the conclusion between the public and the prisoner. (*OB,* Jan. 1801: pp. 95–99)

Woodman and Tidy described the sequence of events as of 1877 when a medical man became involved as a witness:

> The coroner, who is supreme judge in his own court, can issue a summons for the attendance of any legally qualified medical practitioner. You must not, therefore, refuse to go, *merely because* you know nothing about the case. Your opinion may be required as a skilled

witness upon collateral issues of fact or opinion. The ordinary fee for a medical witness is one guinea. . .

Supposing the case in which the inquest has been held ends in a verdict of manslaughter, or murder, you will probably have to appear at a police court, or before magistrates, and you will then be bound over to give evidence on the trial. Of this you will receive due notice. A sum of £20 or £40 is usually named as a penalty for non-attendance. No medical man is bound to attend a trial unless a subpoena has been placed in his hands a reasonable time beforehand. In civil cases a payment of some kind is needed to make the subpoena binding. . . .

A professional witness should ask for and obtain his reasonable expenses; and he is not bound in a civil trial, nor always in a police court, to give evidence until so paid. But when once sworn, he cannot legally refuse to give evidence as to matters of fact. (1877: pp. 24–29)

Advice to the expert witness was proffered by a good many other writers on forensic medicine. John G. Smith told of a surgical friend who "declared that he was never in such a fright in his life, as when summoned" to the witness box. But, said Smith stoutly, "Ignorance is the real parent of this dread" (1825: p. 164). He had a different reason for disliking court appearances:

It is a severe tax upon the time of the practitioner, who, being subpoenaed to give his attendance, has the alternative of being secluded from his patients for several days perhaps, or of forfeiting of £100. Even the remuneration allowed by law is not an equivalent in many instances; for a physician can claim no more than two guineas a day, and this only in civil cases, or when brought forward at the instance of the prosecution. For attending as a witness in behalf of the prisoner in a *criminal* case, although we are equally obliged to go, we are paid nothing. This being the state of such matters, no wonder that lawyers complain of our reluctance to assist them. (1829: p. 12)

Michael Ryan urged his colleagues not to be overwhelmed by counsel. It is, he said,

proverbial that the most eminent members of the [medical] faculty are among the worst witnesses in our courts of justice. This arises from the novelty of their situation, and from the brow-beating and bullying behaviour of rude lawyers, which one would think is caused by a desire to impede, and not to promote, the ends of justice—the elicitation of truth. Medical men should recollect that they hold the same rank in the state as lawyers, are as useful and respectable members of society, and therefore not be insulted and perplexed by the pettifogging scurrility of their rivals, who are often their inferiors in talent. . . . When advocates behave in this manner, they are to be treated with utter contempt, and in no case should a medical man lose his patience or temper. This is the fatal secret which defeats forensic trickery. (1836: p. 460)

Another nineteenth-century writer on forensic medicine was troubled by the seemingly biased position in which expert witnesses may be placed, "for being compelled to appear on the side either of the prosecution or of the defense, they are consequently made to assume more or less of the appearance of partisans—a position derogatory to, and inconsistent with, the dignity and neutrality of science. . . . it is most desirable that all evidence relating to the abstract principles of science, and their application to jurisprudential purposes, should be delivered from neutral ground" (Robinson, 1856: p. 3).

Sensible rules were set down in 1877 for the conduct of the professional witness in court:

> I. Make yourself as fully acquainted as possible with all facts of the case on which you have to give evidence. Let your post-mortem examination be a thorough one. . . . You should also refresh your memory by a reference to some standard work on the subject, so as to know the view held by authorities. . . .
>
> II. Be punctual to the time appointed for the inquiry.
>
> III. Avoid all flippancy of manner. . . .
>
> IV. Arrange what you have to say . . . in a methodical manner. *You cannot be too clear about dates.* It is well to affix the day of the week, as well as that of the month, to every important event. . . .
>
> V. Use the plainest English you can, and never strive to appear learned by the use of scientific or court terms. Let the result of a blow be a *bruise* rather than a contusion; speak of a *blood-clot* rather than of apoplectic extravasation.
>
> VI. Do not answer any question unless you both hear it and clearly understand it; and take care to give your own evidence so as to be heard and understood. Your evidence given in a village inn may be read and commented upon by the medical and legal professions throughout the world.[19]
>
> VII. Never lose your temper in the witness-box. . . .
>
> VIII. Avoid prolixity and useless repetitions. Volunteer as little evidence as possible; but keep back no part of the truth. . . .
>
> IX. Keep your *opinions,* together with all disputed circumstances, quite separate from those *facts* which you have yourself observed, or which are satisfactorily proved by the evidence. . . .
>
> X. Whilst avoiding undue hesitation, as you would avoid undue precipitancy, take time so as to frame your answer that it may convey your real meaning, and be easily understood. . . .
>
> XI. The law is very strict on the point of written notes. The witness is not allowed to read his evidence, although he is allowed to refresh his memory by referring to his notes. Further, all notes referred to in the witness-box must have been made at the time to which they refer; and if the notes themselves are to be admitted as evidence,

19. Coroners' inquests were often held in inns and public houses, which afforded the largest appropriate places of assembly.

they must be the originals, and not copies. . . . Take care that your depositions are read over to you before signing them.

XII. The highest legal authorities have decided that there is no special privilege attaching to medical men with regard to secrets of a professional nature. . . . This is the law; and however it may be defended on legal grounds, we hope that there are many medical men who would prefer to sacrifice their personal liberty to their honour. (1877: pp. 27–28)

The taking of careful notes, particularly at the scene of a crime or at autopsy, seems to have been the exception rather than the rule. Obviously such records were always important, but they were seldom mentioned in testimony except by experienced witnesses like Alfred Swaine Taylor. Many medical experts admitted on the stand that they were obliged to rely on their memories. Thus, for example, the court to a medical witness: "Which side of the head was it upon?—Upon my word, I have almost forgot on which side it was; I think it was on the left, but I am not positive of that" (*OB,* April 1795: pp. 562–602). Or consider the almost visible anguish of a surgeon, trying to remember as counsel for the prosecution relentlessly tightens the screw:

> I have seen and made many *post-mortem* examinations and have taken the ordinary hospital notes—I have not my notes here—I took the headings of the different viscera, and when I got home made out my notes in a small pocket-book, which contains private matters besides, I have searched for that book but cannot find it—the last time I saw it it was in my consulting-room; it is a small book. . . . the notes of the *post-mortem* examination did not occupy very much of the book; perhaps two pages and a half—I do—I do not think I have said before that they occupied much more than that. . . . they were the only notes I made—the book is lost and cannot be found. . . . I have my notes here; my dispenser has them in the bag—they are not an exact copy of the notes in the book that I lost; there is a great addition to them—the set of notes I made half an hour after the examination are on the blue paper. . . . the other set of notes, Dr. Bright's, were made on the Sunday—the post-mortem examination was on the Thursday, I think. . . . the chief part of the post-mortem examination, the dirty part of it, was done by my partner, Mr. Piggott. (*OB,* Sept. 1877: pp. 313–93)

(It is of interest, incidentally, that by the middle of the nineteenth century police officers regularly were able to give precise and clearly expressed testimony.)

Sketches of fatal injuries and the like are seldom mentioned. They would often have been useful, particularly in the years before the introduction of photography into police and forensic science. On the other hand, surveyors who came to the stand to give information as to the construction of a building or the dimensions of a room were well prepared with plans and models.

THE AUTOPSY

Dissection of the human body in order to observe both normal structure and the alterations produced by disease probably began in Alexandria in the third century B.C. Dissections were undertaken in the Middle Ages, sometimes for medicolegal purposes. Detailed written reports of autopsies date from the late fifteenth century, at least for the Continent (King and Meehan, 1973: pp. 518–20, 523; O'Neill, 1976). Kölliker published the first textbook on histology in 1852; Virchow's classic *Cellular Pathology* appeared in 1858. In Britain, systematic post-mortem dissection and the study of morbid anatomy began to come into their own in the latter part of the eighteenth century under the influence of William and John Hunter, Astley Cooper, and Percivall Pott (Long, 1928: p. 156).

Probably the first significant publications in English on pathology were Matthew Baillie's *Morbid Anatomy* (1793; Rodin, 1973) and John Hunter's *A Treatise on the Blood, Inflammation, and Gun-Shot Wounds* (1794). Hunter, an inveterate experimenter, had long studied what we call infection and had had experience with gunshot wounds during his years as an army surgeon. Baillie was a nephew and student of John and William Hunter. His important volume dealt with the pathology of disease, although not that of trauma, and demonstrated the virtues of meticulous observation. Knowledge of gross pathology was advanced in Britain in the first half of the nineteenth century by such major figures as Joseph Hodgson, Richard Bright, Thomas Hodgkin, and Dominic John Corrigan (Mettler, 1947: p. 256), while others contributed to the new field of microscopic pathology (McMenemy, 1968: pp. 18–23). A systematic course in histology was introduced in Edinburgh in the winter of 1841–42 by Hughes Bennett.

But except for geniuses like John Hunter, few men had learned to perform, or understood the value of, a careful medicolegal autopsy. William Dease, writing later on medical jurisprudence, emphasized the particular importance of ascertaining the cause of death in cases of external injury, possible poisoning, and suspected infanticide. A practical knowledge of anatomy was essential, Dease continued, but competent anatomists were rare in the cities and almost nonexistent in the country; "from this defect many dreadful mistakes have been committed, to the scandal of the profession, and irretrievable injury of the person accused" (1819: p. 85). Here was another reason for the slow emergence of forensic medicine. John Gordon Smith complained in 1829:

> I do not believe there is a medical man educated in England who can open a dead body, certainly not one who could name the instruments required to perform this operation—for judiciary purposes unless he may be found among my own pupils, or those of my friend Professor Christison of Edinburgh. Some time ago I offered to instruct certain medical officers how to do this with great advantage and convenience;—but what answer did I receive from their local chief? Why this—That the thing was impracticable according to my plans, and quite out of the question. (1829: pp. 20–21)

Another observer inveighed against the practice of entrusting the post-mortem examination "to persons not qualified for that especial duty—to persons who have not been daily exercised in observation of pathological or morbid change in the structure of the body" (Alderson, 1856).

Permission for an autopsy was infrequently refused. If the procedure was undertaken, internal examination of the body was commonly incomplete or entirely omitted:

> The Skull was not laid open, because it is judg'd to be unnecessary where there was no Bleeding at the Nose, or Ears, no *Comus* [coma?], nor any of the Symptoms of a fracture'd Skull. (*OB*, July 1738; pp. 109–11)

> upon observing the wound at the bottom of the breast, I proposed opening the body several times to the [coroner's] jury, but they thought it needless, they were so well satisfied. (*OB*, Sept. 1745: pp. 218–23)

> Did you open the body at all?—No, there was not the least reason for it, neither do I apprehend I should have got any additional information from opening it. . . .
>
> What appeared to you then from the inspection of the body, to have been the probable cause of her death?—I cannot say. (*OB*, Feb. 1784: pp. 445–57)

> the Coroner asked if we thought a *post mortem* examination necessary, but we had no doubt of death being caused by the fall, and the friends objected to it. (*OB*, July 1838: pp. 512–13)

One autopsy was performed with, it was alleged, completely negative results:

> I made a *post-mortem* examination . . . and could not find anything to account for his death—all the organs were healthy.

> Cross-examined. *Q*. In your opinion, was death caused by fear? *A*. Yes—he fell out of the window 3 feet, and that might have been another cause of death. (*OB*, Sept. 1870: p. 498)

By 1877 a medical man could not

> legally refuse to make a post-mortem examination if the coroner requests it, and you cannot claim more than two guineas for your attendance and the autopsy, including a chemical analysis of the stomach, etc. But if you do not feel competent to make the analysis you ought to say so, and refuse to perform in a hasty and improper manner that which may involve not only the life but the reputation of others. A coroner may ask you to make a post-mortem examination *whilst* the inquest is being held, and by artificial light. You ought to protest against this, as it is impossible to make a careful examination of the whole body in less than an hour, and, if it be possible, daylight is always preferable. The yellow tinge given to the skin by certain poisons (picric acid, *e.g.*), and the same tint produced by disease (*e.g.*, jaundice), may easily escape notice by candle or gaslight. (Woodman and Tidy, 1877: p. 27)

Many trials for homicide were conducted without the benefit of autopsy reports and many more without any expert medical testimony at all. Table 1 summarizes the situation. Autopsy reports for infanticide trials were not included, but all other reports, even of the most perfunctory "the body was opened" type of post-mortem examination, were counted. The large majority of the reports, like most of the other expert medical testimony, was given by surgeons. The steady increase after 1778 in the proportion of homicide trials at which autopsy findings were described reflects the influence of eighteenth-century surgeon-pathologists like Hunter and Cooper, the subsequent appearance of textbooks, and the initiation of university courses dealing with forensic medicine, together with a slowly growing recognition of the essential role of the medical expert. Increasingly such witnesses were called not only by the prosecution but also by the defense.

I

English Forensic Medicine to 1700

As a prelude to a survey of early forensic medicine in England, a short account of the beginnings of this science in the rest of Western Europe will permit a comparison of forensic medical development on both sides of the Channel and a perception of England's curiously slow progress in the field.

THE CONTINENT

The appearance on the Continent of expert medical testimony as part of the legal process cannot be precisely dated,[1] but it is known that the Slavic and Germanic peoples who overran the Roman Empire in the fifth century established the system of *Wehrgeld,* or monetary compensation for wounds or murder, paid to the injured person or to the dead man's relatives. The courts used medical experts to evaluate the severity of the wounds so that the amount of the penalty could be decided. Subsequently, in an effort to regularize legal procedures, codes of laws were drawn up under Charlemagne (782–814), Godfrey de Bouillon in 1100, Roger II of Sicily in 1140, Pope Innocent III in 1209, Pope Gregory IX in 1234, Philip the Bold in 1278, Pope John

1. For extended discussions of early European legal medicine, see Paris and Fonblanque, 1823: pp. ix–xxiv; Cumstom, 1910, 1912; Ackerknecht and Kozelka, 1950; S. Smith, 1951, 1954; Simpson, 1961, 1969a; Camps, 1968: pp. 3–10; Taylor, 1974; Smyth, 1980: pp. 17–22.

XXII in the fourteenth century, and others. The laws and edicts repeatedly instructed the courts to seek medical advice in questions of poisoning, wounding, murder, infanticide, suicide, abortion, pregnancy, legitimacy, impotence, witchcraft, and the diagnosis of leprosy. The doctor could also be involved in the courts' attempts to extract evidence under torture. There are records of medicolegal autopsies of sorts, particularly when poisoning was suspected.

Two important bodies of criminal law were introduced in Germany in the sixteenth century. The *Bambergische Halsgerichtsordnung,* or *Bamberger Code,* of 1507, supplemented and extended by *Constitutio criminalis Carolina,* of Charles V, the *Caroline Code* of 1533, provided for consultation with medical experts in cases of abortion, concealed pregnancy, infanticide, drowning, and medical malpractice; defined suicide as a felony, thus raising medicolegal problems; and called for post-mortem examination after a violent death and for medical determination of the sanity or insanity of the accused. It is Ackerknecht's belief that the "greatest single accomplishment of medical men in the field of legal medicine in this period was their fight against the superstitious belief in witchcraft and sorcery which annually sent thousands of mentally ill persons to the stake" (Ackerknecht and Kozelka, 1950; p. 1290). Led by a fearless Dutchman, Jan Wier, or Weyer, a small group of physicians battled against unreasoning prejudice toward the insane and helped to establish the fundamental legal principle that such persons may not be responsible for their actions.

The first book on forensic medicine was probably that of the great French surgeon, Ambroise Paré, in 1575 (*Oeuvres*). Translated into English, the little treatise, *How to Make Reports, and to Embalme the Dead* (1634), is full of sound advice and information on the responsibilities of the surgeon in determining the cause of violent death, on tests for virginity and pregnancy, and other matters. Paré describes the steps that should be taken "if it chance that a nurse either through drunkennesse, or negligence, lyes upon her infant lying in bed with her, and so stifles or smothers it to death. If your judgement be required, whether the infant dyed through the default, or negligence of the nurse? or through some violent or suddaine diseases that lay hidden and lurking in the body thereof?" (Parey, 1634: p. 1124). The surgeon then tells how the cause of death can be determined.

Paré's treatise includes several case studies, among them one of an almost fatal suffocation by what we would recognize as carbon monoxide, "the vapour of kindled or burning charcoales" in a closed room, and a perceptive description of the signs of drowning:

"Whosoever is found dead in the waters, you shall know whether they were throwne into the water alive or dead. For all the belly of him that was throwne in alive, will be swollen, and puffed up by reason of the water that is contained therein; certaine clammie excrements come out at his mouth and nosethrills, the ends of his fingers will be worne and excoriated, because that hee dyed striving and digging or scraping in the sand or bottome of the river, seeking somewhat whereon hee might take hold to save himselfe from drowning." (Parey, 1634: p. 1125).

About two decades later there appeared the *Methodus testificandi* of Baptista Condronchi (1597), which discussed legal aspects of wounds, puberty, virginity, pregnancy, labor, poisoning, and sudden death. A more important work on legal medicine was the *De relationibus medicorum* by the Italian Fortunato Fideli. Printed in 1602, the book treats of wounds, smothering, strangling, virginity, malpractice, and other matters. Still another volume on legal medicine, *Medicus politicus* (The political doctor), was published by Roderigo de Castro in 1614.

Paolo Zacchia's massive and comprehensive *Quaestiones medicolegales* earned its author recognition as "the father of legal medicine" (Ackerknecht and Kozelka, 1950: p. 1292). The first seven volumes appeared between 1621 and 1635, the eighth and ninth in 1666. The talented Zacchia, trained in law as well as medicine, was physician to Popes Innocent X and Alexander VII and had lengthy service in the Rota Romana, the papal court of final appeals. He dealt systematically and fully with such problems as the definition of insanity, the determination of fetal age, rape, death during childbirth, malingering, torture, miracles, and witchcraft. Zacchia—and his successors for a long time afterward—were greatly handicapped in detecting poisons by the lack of specific and reliable chemical tests; the investigator was compelled to rely on such uncertain criteria as the appearance of organs, the taste and smell of a suspected substance, and trials of the latter in animals. Zacchia's consideration of several problems was influenced by his experience in the papal court. Impotence, for example, might be alleged as the basis for seeking annulment of a marriage by the Church. Other justification for annulment might be a disease such as leprosy; its diagnosis could result in a medicolegal problem. Zacchia also included in his great work an extensive discussion of public health, at that time and until the nineteenth century often included in the field of legal medicine.

The first organized series of lectures on medicine in relation to law was given in 1650 by Michaelis at the University of Leipzig (Camps,

1968: p. 9). The same city saw the publication ten years later of *Rationale vulnerum letalium judicium* (The rational investigation of deadly wounds), by G. Welsch (1660); in it he recommended procedures for medicolegal autopsies. Not long afterward Johannes Bohn lectured in Leipzig on legal medicine. His *De renunciatione vulnerum* (On the reporting of wounds, 1689), discussed their varieties, distinguishing between those received before and those after death and describing also the effects of strangulation and drowning. Special mention should be made of Théophile Bonet, who in 1679 published the details of his findings in nearly three thousand autopsies and demonstrated the great importance of the post-mortem examination (Bonet, 1679).

Valentini's *Corpus juris medico-legale* (1722), embodying two of his works produced earlier in the eighteenth century, and J. F. Zittman's *Medicina forensis* (1706) reviewed series of medicolegal cases and questions raised in German courts. H. F. Teichmeyer's *Institutiones medicinae legalis* (1723) became an important textbook.[2] Of great influence was G. B. Morgagni's *De sedibus et causis morborum* (On the seats and causes of diseases, 1761). A landmark in the history of pathology, it consisted of a series of letters written over twenty years and based on more than six hundred dissections; included were studies of drowning, strangulation, and hanging.

Other notable contributions were those of Antoine Louis and F. E. Fodéré, a surgeon to Napoleon. The former wrote on, among other subjects, the maximum duration of human pregnancy (1764). In some cases of disputed legitimacy, the courts had accepted claims that pregnancies could last thirteen or fourteen months; Louis attacked this ancient error. Fodéré's *Les Lois éclairées par les sciences physiques* (1798) was the first treatise on forensic medicine to appear in France since the time of Paré (Cumston, 1910). A journal of legal medicine was founded in Berlin in 1782, and late in the same century professorships in the subject were established in Paris, Strasbourg, and Montpellier (Camps, 1968: p. 9).

In considering the development of Continental legal medicine, one is struck by the seemingly prompt recognition of its importance and utility. The lines of scholarly communication were open. Jurists conceded that in certain circumstances they needed to seek outside their own specialty for expert medical advice and information and that the obvious source was the medical man. Final determination of the de-

2. The distinguished physiologist Albrecht von Haller was Teichmeyer's son-in-law.

gree of guilt and responsibility under criminal law remained in the hands of the court, but it was recognized that in certain kinds of cases the decision might depend on medical knowledge and opinion. The establishment of legal codes provided guidance and directions as to when and how expert professional assistance should be sought.

As legal precedents and guidelines developed, so did medicolegal experience. Periodically, doctors also familiar with the law, men like Zacchia and Valentini, were able to extend medicolegal knowledge and practice and to record for the benefit of others what had been learned. Very slowly, a healthy medical skepticism developed, helping to erode much of the superstition and prejudice still in evidence in courts of law. The crucial importance of the medicolegal autopsy and of careful medical records was gradually recognized.

The development of legal medicine was of course limited by the fact that it could be understood only by those who read Latin. With the notable exception of Paré's little treatise on *Reports*—like his other works written originally in French for the benefit of his fellow barber surgeons—most Continental books on legal medicine were in Latin until the middle of the eighteenth century, which put them beyond the reach of many surgeons and most barber surgeons. Of little education, these men had learned their skills as apprentices and sometimes, if they were fortunate, from lectures in the vernacular. Existing knowledge of legal medicine was beyond their reach even if they desired it.

ENGLAND

In England the theory and practice of medicine in relation to law lagged far behind that on the Continent, a situation that was to prevail until the nineteenth century.[3] English legal medicine did not enjoy the recognition and regularization of a Carolinian Code, although passages in Bracton indicate that some elements of forensic medicine existed in Britain as early as the thirteenth century (Thorne, 1968: *2*, 1201). It is not quite true that, as Flower asserts, no medical profession existed in England at this time (1944: p. 380), but medical knowledge was certainly primitive. For example, when it was alleged in 1220 that

3. J. G. Smith, 1829: p. 6; Cummin, 1833; Ackerknecht and Kozelka, 1950: p. 1298.

a young man had become a leper,[4] the court turned to a panel of barons of the exchequer for an expert opinion (*Curia regis,* 1938: *8,* 308–09; Flower, 1944: p. 309). Presumably their opinion was considered more valid than that of any available medical practitioner. In separate legal cases in 1221, 1222, and 1223 it was claimed that women rather recently widowed were pregnant; a question of property inheritance made expert opinion particularly important in two of these actions. Each time the court assembled a panel of "worthy matrons" and instructed them to determine by palpation of the breasts and abdomen whether pregnancy existed (Maitland, 1887: *2,* 161–62; *3,* 417–18, 473; Flower, 1944: p. 380); perhaps some of the matrons were midwives. In 1282 a coroner needed to know whether a man struck by an arrow in the breast would die; the opinion of a highly regarded surgeon was sought. In his judgment the patient could not survive (Sayles, 1936: p. 126). (This last, incidentally, appears to be the earliest example of expert surgical opinion rendered in England for a medicolegal reason.)

In January 1299 the rector of a London parish, one William, got into trouble with the law because he had had the decaying carcasses of four wolves sent to him from the Continent (Bartsch, 1920: p. 444). William said they were needed to treat "Le Lou," Old French for *loup* (wolf). This tuberculous disease of the skin is still known as *lupus,* Latin for wolf, a term originating perhaps because the malady can cause scars suggesting a wolf's bite. In accord with the medical doctrine of *similia similibus curantur* (like things are cured by like things), the wolves' flesh would no doubt have been eaten or applied to the lesions to relieve them. William at first claimed that he was a victim of the disease and that this was why he had purchased the bodies. But when questioned by the mayor and aldermen of London, he finally admitted that he did not have lupus or know anyone who did. Furthermore, he confessed that he was not a medical man and therefore was not qualified to treat the malady anyway. At this point the sheriffs were instructed to call into court on an appointed day all of the physicians and surgeons of the City of London, a formidable panel indeed. After consultation, the experts testified that their learned manuscripts did not prescribe wolf flesh for the treatment of any disease (Thomas, 1924: p. 51).

4. In medieval times the term *leprosy* was used imprecisely to describe some forms of syphilis and other afflictions as well (Creighton, 1965: *1,* 70–79).

Surgical malpractice suits began cropping up in fourteenth-century legal documents.[5] Curiously enough, although questions of surgical skill and judgment were central, the court often depended entirely on lay testimony, the issue being whether, not why, a surgeon had failed to cure his patient. But sometimes, as in February 1354, an issue of professional competence was raised. Under oath before the mayor, aldermen, and sheriffs of London, four surgeons, one of them also the prior of a French monastery,[6] were called on to testify

> as to a certain enormous and terrible hurt, on the right side of the jaw of Thomas de Shene appearing, whether or not such injury was curable at the time when John le Spicer of Cornhulle took the same Thomas under his care.
>
> Who say upon their oath, that if the aforesaide John le Spicer, at the time when he took the said Thomas under his care, had been expert in his art or craft, or had called in counsel and assistance to his aid, he might have cured the injury aforesaid; and they further say that, through want of skill on the part of the said John le Spicer, the said injury under his care has become apparently incurable.[7]

Malpractice was again the issue in February 1377. One Richard Cheyndut had been entrusted with the care of a boy's diseased leg. As a result of Cheyndut's alleged carelessness and ignorance, the youth was likely to lose his limb. By order of the mayor, three surgeons examined the patient. In their opinion, "it would require great experience, care and expense if the leg were to be cured without permanent injury." Damages were awarded to the plaintiff (Thomas, 1929: p. 236; Cosman, 1972, 1973).

Astrology was an important element in medical practice, for it was widely believed that the heavenly bodies helped to regulate human temperament, destiny, and health and disease. Drawings of "zodiacal man" showed which planet controlled each part of the body; the surgeon dared not ignore his patient's horoscope. When on 31 January 1424 a certain William Forest received a serious wound in the muscles of his right thumb, it was observed that the moon was "consumed in a bloody sign, to wit, Aquarius, under a very malevolent constellation." Ten days later, when the moon was in the sign of Gemini, the wound bled dangerously. Three different barber surgeons undertook

5. Records survive for at least a dozen of these cases in the fourteenth century and for another ten in the fifteenth. Some have been discussed by Cosman, 1972, 1973; and Chapman, 1982.

6. He may have been a prisoner of war in England. It was not unusual for members of certain religious orders to practice medicine.

7. Riley, 1868: pp. 273–74; Rogers, 1891: p. 5; Cosman, 1973.

to stop the hemorrhage, which broke out six times. Finally, fearful of Forest's death from loss of blood, one of the surgeons obtained his patient's consent to check the flow by applying a hot iron, "as was proper, and thus saved his life." But, as had been anticipated, the hand was mutilated. Eight physicians and surgeons were called in by the court to arbitrate the question of alleged error in Forest's treatment. It was their expert decision on 9 June 1424 that the barber surgeons had acted correctly. Not only were they absolved, but perpetual silence in the matter was enjoined upon the plaintiff, and the good reputation of the defendants was to be restored as fully as possible. In the opinion of the learned consultants, "any defect, mutilation or disfigurement of the hand was due either to the constellation aforesaid, or some defect of the patient, or the original nature of the wound" (Thomas, 1943: pp. 174–75; Cosman, 1972, 1973).

A panel of lay persons, this time not barons but "discreet and law abiding" citizens, was called in October 1420 to decide whether a certain man was a leper; if he were, a writ would be issued obliging him forever to shun the company of others (Sayles, 1971: p. 247). Once again, in the face of what we would consider an eminently medical problem, the officers of the law chose to rely on the opinion of respected laymen rather than to consult the doctors. Anyone, it was implied, could recognize leprosy; in this grave situation the *probity* of the witnesses was the important consideration.

In fifteenth-century England the reliability and prestige of medical knowledge as such were still on very uncertain ground. The physician limited his observations mostly to a study of pulse and urine; the surgeon, much lower in the professional scale, was guided only by the most obvious manifestations of injury and malfunction. Both practitioners depended heavily for guidance on tradition, ancient writings, and the precepts of astrology. True medical science, daring to move ahead on the strength of its own discoveries and proofs, was yet to come. It follows that forensic medicine was in an even more undeveloped state.

But judges continued on occasion to seek medical assistance, as in September 1468, when doctors were ordered to determine whether a woman, Joan de Nightyngale, was suffering from leprosy. They decided that she was free of four different forms of the disease.[8] Expert opinion of sorts was required in a contested inheritance case in 1696.

8. Rymer, 1710: *11*, 635–36; A suspected case, 1940: *2*, 441; Calendar, 1953: *2*, 30–31.

We are told that a certain "Sir Francis Willoughby died Seized of a great Inheritance, having five daughters, whereof the eldest was married to Perc[ival] Willoughby and not any Sons; And the said Sir Francis, leaving his wife Dorothy, who at the time of his death, pretended her self to be with Child by Sir Francis, which if it were a Son, all the five Sisters should therby lose the Inheritance descended unto them." Naturally this came as unwelcome news to the survivors. Percival and his wife Bridget obtained a writ *de ventre inspiciendo* from the Court of Chancery that would cause Dorothy "to be viewed by twelve knights, and searched by twelve Women in the presence of the twelve knights" to determine whether she were pregnant. If so, the searchers, who may have been midwives, were to certify how long it would be until she would deliver her child. They reported that she was twenty weeks pregnant. Now another writ was issued directing that Dorothy be kept in a well-guarded house under daily surveillance by some of the matrons. They were to observe the delivery and learn whether the child was male or female, "to the intent there should not be any Falsity." The unfortunate Dorothy sat out the remaining months of her confinement, finally went into labor, and produced—a daughter (Grimston, 1683a: *1*, 566).

Expert testimony was required in another inheritance case in 1619. A certain Edward Andrews had died of plague on 23 March 1610. His widow was delivered of a baby daughter on 5 January 1611, "forty weeks and nine days later." For six weeks before the birth the pregnant woman had been harrassed by her father-in-law, who "did much abuse her, and caused her to be dislodged from places where she was harboured, and to lie in the cold Streets." More trouble came to mother and daughter in 1619, when a legal action was brought to determine whether the little girl, born in 1611, was indeed the child of the deceased Edmund Andrews and thus could inherit, or whether she was illegitimate. Opinions were sought from

> two Doctors of Physick, *viz.* Sir *William Baddy* and Doctor Mundford, and one *Chamberlaine* (who was a physician, and in nature of a Midwife)[9] upon their Oath, they affirming that the child came in time convenient to be the Daughter of the party who died; And that the usual time for a Woman to go with child, was nine months and ten days, viz. *menses Solares,* that is thirty days to the month, and not

9. "Chamberlaine" was Peter Chamberlen the younger (1572–1626) or Peter Chamberlen the elder (d. 1631), his elder brother, members of a famous family of accoucheurs and proprietors of the Chamberlen obstetrical forceps.

> *menses Lunares,*[10] and that by reason of the want of strength in the woman or the child, or by reason of ill usage, she might be a longer time, *viz,* to the end of ten months, or more. The Court held here, that it might well be as the Physicians had affirmed, that ten months may be said properly to be the time *mulieribus pariendo constitutum.*[11]

A legal argument ensued, and cases were cited on both sides of the question, but the judge was not to be swayed. The most remarkable precedent invoked was that of a woman in Paris who allegedly delivered her husband's child fourteen months after his death (Grimston, 1683b: pp. 541–42).

One can scarcely omit from this series of early medicolegal opinions the report of William Harvey, the discoverer of the circulation, on his autopsy on 16 November 1635 on the body of Thomas Parr. Harvey's expert medical opinion as to the cause of death was requested by Charles I. As Keele points out, the autopsy was made in exemplary fashion (1965: pp. 90–91). Although probably not the first post-mortem examination in England, it is the earliest for which I have found a record.

Parr had died on 14 November at the alleged age of 152 years and nine months. Not long before his demise, the old man had been brought to London by the Earl of Arundel and introduced to King Charles. When Parr had breathed his last, the monarch, like everyone else, wondered how death had been so long held at bay. Harvey, in company with several other leading physicians, found both the exterior of the body and the internal organs, except the lungs, to be sound and healthy. He added in awe that

> it seemed not improbable that the common report was true, viz. that he did public penance under a conviction for [sexual] incontinence after he had passed his hundredth year; and his wife, whome he had married as a widow in his hundred-and-twentieth year, did not deny that he had intercourse with her after the manner of other husbands with their wives.

Parr's diet had been

> sub-rancid cheese, milk in every form, coarse and hard bread, and small drink, generally sour whey. On this sorry fare, but living in his home, free from care, did this poor man attain to such length of days. He even ate something about midnight shortly before his death.

10. Lunar months of twenty-eight days each.
11. Recognized as usual for pregnancy in women.

The latter was ascribed by Harvey to what we would call pneumonia, brought on when he left the pure air of the country for London,

> a city whose grand characteristic is an immense concourse of men and animals, and where ditches abound, and filth and offal lie scattered about, to say nothing of the smoke engendered by the general use of sulphureoús coal as fuel, whereby the air is at all times rendered heavy, but much more so in the autumn that at any other season. (Willis, 1847: pp. 587–92; Keele: pp. 37–38, 90–91)

Environmental pollution is not a recent problem.

We come now to what seems to be the first recorded English homicide trial at which expert medical testimony was heard and to what must have been one of the first medicolegal autopsies in England.

The Earl of Pembroke was tried in 1678 by a jury of his peers for the murder of Nathaniel Cony. It was alleged that the earl had kicked Cony in the belly. Post-mortem examination showed large bruises and a quantity of extravasated blood in the abdomen. At the trial four surgeons and two physicians were called to testify; both of the latter had attended Cony before his death, and the surgeons and one of the physicians, Dr. Conquest, had been present at the autopsy. The other, Dr. Lower, had sought not to become involved in the post-mortem examination,[12] explaining that "I was desired to be present at the dissection, but because of the rumor of this business [the homicide charge], I said it would be a troublesome matter, and therefore would purposely avoid it."

Expert medical opinion was sought by the court in relation to two questions. What caused the internal hemorrhage? Was it fatal? It developed that Cony was a hard drinker. According to his doctors, he had not complained to them of being kicked or beaten. Mr. Raven, one of the surgeons at the autopsy, testified that he saw no bruises but did find clotted blood in the abdomen: "This blood, I think, my lord, must be extravasated by the violence of his gripes, for it is proved he drank a great quantity of claret, and afterwards of small-beer, which set the blood upon a fermentation, that set him vomiting; by the violence thereby used to nature this blood was thrown down into the belly."

It is notable that the autopsy did not extend to examination of the

12. Richard Lower (1631–91), a distinguished physiologist and anatomist and the most noted London physician of his time, in 1665 was the first to transfuse blood directly from one animal to another.

viscera for injuries that could have caused the hemorrhage. Instead, a convenient medical theory was invoked in explanation of the death. In his summing up, the judge reminded the jury that "we are to enquire, whether he [Cony] came to his death by those blows given him by the prisoner at the bar." The jury seems to have rejected the surgeon's theory; the Earl of Pembroke was found guilty of manslaughter (Howell, 1816: *6*, 1309–50).

The next year three men were tried for the killing of Sir Edmundbury Godfrey. It was alleged that they and others had strangled him with a twisted handkerchief. The body was found "in a ditch, with his sword through him, and the end of it two handfuls out of his back . . . but there was no blood at all when it was taken out." Post-mortem examination showed severe bruising, two stab wounds of the chest, and dislocation of the neck. Skillard, the autopsy surgeon, noted that a sword had passed through the thorax and heart. But, he said, these wounds had not killed Sir Edmundbury, since they had not bled. Furthermore, the shirt and waistcoat he was wearing, only partly fastened, had not been pierced by a sword. In other words, the body had been wounded after death, and then had been incompletely dressed.

Since it was established that the victim's neck had been either broken or dislocated, the Attorney General asked whether it was possible, as rumored, that Sir Edmundbury might have hanged himself and that his relatives had thereafter run him through with a sword "to save his estate." This raised an important legal point; if Sir Edmundbury while of sound mind had committed suicide, he would be accounted a felon and all his possessions would be forfeit to the Crown. But Skillard was convinced that the cervical dislocation was caused by more violence than a suicidal hanging (Howell, 1816: 1, cols. 184–85).

On 13 March 1699 the corpse of a girl, Sarah Stout, spinster, was found floating in a mill pond. The body was buried, but subsequently suspicion developed that Sarah had been murdered. In addition, the girl's mother was disturbed by reports that her daughter had been pregnant. So on 28 April, six weeks later, the remains were exhumed and a post-mortem examination was performed by a group of prominent London surgeons and physicians including William Cowper, anatomist; Sir Samuel Garth, successful physician and literary and political figure; and Sir Hans Sloane, distinguished physician and collector, founder, ultimately secretary, and then president of the Royal Society, and first physician to be created a baronet. Much was made of the fact that the body was found floating in the pond; drowned bodies were known first to sink, an observation that was confirmed by the testimony of two Royal Navy sailors.

A surgeon stated that upon post-mortem examination the body was full of gas but was not putrefied. It contained no water. The uterus showed no sign of conception. It was concluded that the girl had not drowned, since "we found no water in her; her intestines were not putrified; for if there had been water in her, that would have caused a fermentation, and that would have rotted the lungs and guts." The cause of Sarah Stout's death was not established, and the prisoner in the dock was found not guilty (Howell, 1816: 13, col. 1123–36; S. Smith, 1951; p. 604; Rosenberg, 1957; Mant, 1977).

In considering these examples of expert medical testimony elicited by English courts up to the latter part of the seventeenth century, one must bear in mind that, with the single exception of the Johnson translation of Paré's little French treatise in 1634, *no* work in English on forensic medicine had yet been published, or indeed was to appear for many years. No doubt some of the British physicians who could read Latin had encountered Continental works on legal medicine. But the impact of such knowledge seems to have been slight. The first significant and original English writing on forensic medicine was William Hunter's landmark monograph in 1783.

On the other hand, as we have seen, the principle of seeking expert information and opinion for the assistance of the court had been established in England in the Middle Ages. The use of such assistance appears to have been elective, and its importance seems often to have gone unappreciated. Even in the seventeenth century one finds few English trials in which medical men testified.[13] Medicolegal autopsies were the exception rather than the rule until the early nineteenth century.

13. Commented Chaillé in 1876, "Great Britain transmitted to this nation [the United States] laws, barbarously conspicuous for the absence of provisions to apply medical knowledge to the administration of justice, and Anglo-American law continues to be, in large measure, hostile to Medical Jurisprudence" (p. 400).

II

Injuries from Sharp and Blunt Instruments

UNDER ENGLISH LAW A CORONER HAS LONG BEEN OBLIGATED TO investigate by means of an inquest any sudden, violent, or suspicious death occurring in his jurisdiction. Nowadays the duties of the coroner and his jury are identification of the deceased, certification as to when and where death occurred, recording of the medical conditions that led to death, and establishment of the circumstances of death. The expert medical witness, whether appearing before a coroner or a trial judge, is and was well advised to confine himself essentially to two points: when did death occur and what medical conditions caused it? Much of the science of forensic medicine has developed from efforts to answer these apparently simple questions.

In medieval times the law required that at an inquest a witness, usually a medical man, report the length and depth of any wound to the coroner's court, which rarely considered the information further. Nevertheless, it was gradually realized by those few who thought about such matters that the nature and appearance of a slash or bruise might tell quite a lot about the weapon, how it had been used, where the assailant had stood when he struck, and other details of potential importance when and if the crime was reconstructed. If at a subsequent trial for homicide some observant medical man established just how and when and where the attack had occurred, the judge and jury were much closer to determining the guilt or innocence of the accused. Clearly the role of the expert medical witness could be of great importance.

British textbook writers at first largely failed to recognize the forensic medical significance of wounds. George Edward Male dealt with them briefly and generally:

> It is necessary to discover by what weapon or instrument a wound has been inflicted; and if the person is dead, or senseless, whether it has been given by himself or another; if any weapon is found near the deceased, we should ascertain if that could possibly have been the cause of the injury or whether it has been placed there afterwards. (Male, 1819: pp. 179–80)

Paris and Fonblanque in their *Medical Jurisprudence* (1823) devote more space to the nature, prognosis, and treatment of various kinds of wounds than to the possible forensic importance of such injuries. However, these authors do point out that the "direction of a wound is frequently a circumstance of much greater importance than may at first appear" (*3,* 119). Ryan's discussion of "contusions, wounds, and homicide by them" (1831: p. 191) also has much more the quality of an elementary textbook on surgical care than of a work on forensic medicine. Guy does discuss incised and other wounds with some perception; for example, "In a recent incised wound, inflicted during life, the edges are everted, the cellular tissue is filled with blood, and there are coagula between the lips of the wound" (1845: p. 301). Guy also considers experiments of Orfila and Taylor on post-mortem wounds in dogs.[1]

WHAT KIND OF WEAPON WAS USED?

Some weapons produced distinctive wounds. At a seventeenth-century homicide trial two surgical witnesses stated that the fatal wound was produced by the prisoner's scimitar, but a third surgeon noted that the wound was triangular in outline and had therefore been inflicted with a rapier (*OB,* Oct. 1685: p. 3). A small carpenter's gouge caused a chest wound "about a quarter of an inch diameter, like a half-moon or curve" (*OB,* Oct. 1755: p. 344). A cooper's howel, used to smooth the inside of a cask and having the end of the plane iron rounded, resulted in a somewhat similar but larger injury (*OB,* July

1. M. J. B. Orfila, a naturalized Spaniard, was founder and dean of the Académie de Médecine in Paris, physician to Louis XVIII, a leader in French forensic medicine, and a popular teacher. He is best known for his book on toxicology, *Traité des poisons* (1814–15), and for studies on post-mortem bleeding (Ackerknecht, 1950: p. 1300).

1708: pp. 2–3). Triangular wounds in a dead woman were allegedly produced by a sharp-ended file (*OB,* Jan. 1852: p. 303).

Not only the shape but the size of the injury were important. A surgeon found a chest wound "into the left ventricle of the heart. . . . I put this knife into the wound, and it fitted exactly" (*OB,* May 1745: p. 170). Another surgeon recognized an important characteristic that could make more difficult the relating of a weapon to a stab wound.

> *Q.* Will not the scissors make a wider wound?
>
> *Saul.* Yes; but the skin will contract after the instrument is drawn out . . . it [the blade of the scissors] was not a double-edged instrument; if it had been, it would have made a broad wound. I do not imagine the orifice could have been broader than the edge of the point; it [the blade of the scissors] is not like a broad-edged tool. (*OB,* Dec. 1760: pp. 18–19)

That is, the dull edge of the scissors blade stretched the skin rather than cutting it; when the blade was withdrawn, the elasticity of the skin caused contraction of the opening.

The *depth* of a penetrating wound was not necessarily equal to the length of the blade which produced the wound. A ship's surgeon, for example, was not sure that a stab wound in a sailor was effected by a knife which the surgeon was shown in court, pointing out that a blade driven hard against the yielding abdominal wall would compress soft structures and penetrate very deeply (*OB,* Oct. 1760: p. 14).

Scratches from human fingernails were distinctive and different from the lacerations produced by claws: "The scratches were down the face, about the width of a finger nail; that was why I said it was a human cat" (*OB,* April 1858: p. 562).

HOW WAS THE WEAPON USED?

Defense wounds, as they are now called, occurred when the victim was trying to protect himself or herself from attack with a sharp weapon, either by grasping it (cuts on flexor surface of hand) or by trying to ward it off (cuts on dorsal surface of hand) (Adelson, 1974; pp. 352–53). The correct interpretation of the angle at which a knife or sword caused a defense wound might help to identify the assailant. In July 1760 one William Robinson, involved in a quarrel while standing on the highway, was attacked with a hanger, a short, slightly curved sword popular with sailors, in the hand of a man on horseback.

Robinson's wrist was slashed on its inner surface from the forearm toward the fingers. Eleven days later he died of a violent fever, undoubtedly occasioned by infection of his wound.

Two days before his death, Robinson had deposed in the court of Sir John Fielding, the famous blind magistrate, that his attacker had given him "a Cutt with his Hanger upon his right Arm as he [Robinson] held it up to Defend his Head." But at the trial of William Roberts for causing Robinson's death, the prosecution claimed that, instead, Robinson's right arm had been in a low position because he was thrusting out aggressively with a stick or was about to seize the bridle of Roberts's horse. Dr. William Hunter, distinguished anatomist, physician, accoucheur, and a friend of William Pitt the Elder, Robinson's employer, resolved the matter when he testified at the trial that Robinson's arm was "cut slanting toward the fingers; it could not be cut as his hand was up, for if so, [the wound] would have been slanting towards his body; it must be while his hand was down, or holding the [Roberts's] horse's bridle" (*OB,* July 1760: pp. 221–38; Inquest, 1760; Forbes, 1976a). So the dead man had deposed falsely.

Late one night in 1839 five men were walking home on a highway from a public house. They had been drinking most of the day and evening. One of them, Aspland, who was very lame, was being carried piggyback by his friend Rashbrook: "my arms were around his neck, and his arms behind me holding me on his back." Aspland later testified that suddenly Rashbrook fell to the ground with his burden, got up, and cried out that he had been stabbed. Bull, another member of the group, ran in panic from the scene and was promptly arrested by the police for the assault on Rashbrook, who died in a few minutes. Bull turned over a bloody knife to a constable and said that he had done the stabbing in self-defense when attacked by Rashbrook.

At Bull's trial, the other men in the group agreed that Rashbrook had been stabbed, not while he was grappling with Bull but while he was carrying Aspland piggyback. The obvious question was, who was telling the truth? Mr. John Hawthorn, a surgeon who had attended the dying Rashbrook and had later performed an autopsy, testified that the great vessels above the armpit were divided, causing a swift and fatal hemorrhage. The pectoral muscle on the front of the chest was not injured. The large axillary vessels could only have been severed if the arm were raised horizontally from the side of the body. So Aspland and his friend were lying (*OB,* Feb. 1839: pp. 539–54).

In defense of a prisoner accused of homicide it might be argued by counsel that the deceased had taken his or her own life. During a trial in 1763 this explanation was offered for the death of a man found with his throat cut. But a surgeon testified that the injury could not have been self-inflicted because the victim also had a fractured skull; after such an injury he could not, the surgeon believed, have slashed his own throat (*OB,* Feb. 1763: p. 106).

In September 1867 John Wiggins was tried in the Old Bailey for the murder of Agnes Oaks. A leading witness was Alfred Swaine Taylor, the distinguished expert on forensic medicine. Wiggins alleged that Agnes Oaks had first tried to slash his throat and then her own. A surgeon said that the woman's throat was cut in such a way that death would have been almost immediate. "The facts consistent with a suicidal infliction of the wound were, that the deceased woman was right-handed, that the wound was situated on the left side of the neck, and its direction was from above downward and from left to right" (Taylor, 1869: p. 497). Inconsistent with the claim of suicide were the facts that the wound began as a stab toward the vertebral column; that, although death must have been instantaneous, her body was found partly under a chair, where it could only have been placed by another person; and that after the wound was produced the woman could not have thrown or placed the knife on a table standing at some distance from where the weapon was found.

The indications were that Wiggins had killed the woman and then had inflicted the wound on his own neck. He alleged that she had slashed him while he was lying down and she was seated behind him. However, said an expert witness, the injury "is superficial like all wounds self-inflicted and imputed to the acts of other persons" (p. 498). There were also major inconsistencies relating to the time at which the prisoner claimed to have found the body, to cuts in the handkerchief he had tied over his neck wound, and so on. Wiggins was sentenced to death (*OB,* Sept. 1867: pp. 509–37; Taylor, 1869). Simpson, reviewing Taylor's observations, comments that in his own experience between 1936 and 1966, "among many hundreds of cut throats there lie only nine that were homicides" (Taylor, 1969 reprint: p. 517).

When death seemed to have been caused by a sharp instrument, it was most unusual for any question to arise as to whether disease might have been a contributing factor. The cause of death was considered self-evident and an autopsy was nearly always dispensed with. This was particularly common before the nineteenth century. Yet illness existing at the time of an attack might actually be the cause of death. On the other hand, fatal sickness once was falsely alleged in defense of an accused.

A man was stabbed with a sword in 1707 and died. His assailant was identified mysteriously as G—— C——. Several surgeons gave evidence that the victim "was poxt [syphilitic], and most of his bowels wasted and rotten." The jury acquitted the accused, stating that his victim "died Visitatione Dei"[2] (*OB,* April 1707: p. 4). Seven years later a man was knifed in the chest; this time the attacker was referred to in the *Sessions Papers* as C——G——. "There were two Surgeons who open'd his Body, and depos'd he did not die of the Wound, for that it had not penetrated the Trunk of the Body; and that he had been an infirm Man for a great while before" (*OB,* Sept. 1714: pp. 4–5). The similarities in these two cases are striking enough to make one wonder. Was the mysterious G——C——, or C——G——, an influential figure, perhaps a nobleman, with a short temper and a purse long enough to bribe the surgeons? In any case, he was found not guilty, both times.

Abdominal injuries were inflicted by a variety of blunt objects, including boots and shoes. Falls or kicks might result in renal trauma or a ruptured spleen. It was observed that a kick in the abdomen could result in a fatal injury without leaving a visible sign. On the other hand, when a woman allegedly was kicked and stamped to death by her husband after he had stabbed her and thrown her downstairs, the surgeon who made the post-mortem examination found nine broken ribs:

> I observ'd something farther, which was very particular. There was one Rib in the Middle of the broken ones, that was not fractured at all; which convinced me, that the rest were broken at several Times, and I imagine with the Heel of his Shoe: for if those that were broke, had been fractur'd by any Instrument, which would break more than one at a Time, it would have been almost impossible that this single Rib should have remained unhurt in the Middle of the fractur'd ones. (*OB,* Sept. 1737: p. 170)

The assailant was sentenced to death.

It was not unusual in homicide trials for disputes to arise over whether death was due to an attack by the accused or to an accidental fall of the victim. We shall encounter this classic forensic problem in

2. *Ex visitatione Dei,* "by the visitation of God." For a discussion of this exculpatory verdict, frequently rendered by coroners' juries, see Forbes, 1978: pp. 7, 32.

many forms. For example, two drunken women fought in the street. The victim allegedly was hit in the face several times with a large key. Later she fell, perhaps striking her face on a curb stone. An observant surgeon found that

> her nose was cut across, at least it was divided—the bridge was broken, and her lip divided in two places—they were contused wounds, not such as a person would receive by a fall in the street—there are three distinct wounds—the one across the nose is a transverse one, the other longitudinal, and the other oblique—the cut on the upper lip was oblique and flat over, so that the force must have been applied upwards, and there is an excoriation on the nose upwards, which would not occur in a fall. . . . the wounds correspond with the key, and the key is stained with blood now.
>
> *Cross-examined. Q.* If a person fell against the curb-stone, might not that cut the lip, and break the teeth? *A.* Not in that way . . . the wounds were all in different directions. (*OB,* April 1840: pp. 981–83)

A blunt instrument sometimes caused an apparently incised injury. In 1864 a man who had been robbed and later was found semiconscious in the street was thought to have been struck on the head with an iron bar, yet the surgeon who attended him before his death found three transverse cuts and a depressed fracture of the skull, all on the back of the head. Laboratory experiments with cadavers, most unusual until the nineteenth century, provided an answer.

> DR. RANDALL. I am a graduate of the University of London . . . I performed several experiments with an instrument like this, with a view to prove that it was not done by this instrument, but we produced three wounds of exactly the same character, on similar matter, not on a living subject. . . . the result of my experiments has been to satisfy me that a wedge with an edge formed by a surface such as this would produce these wounds—this is a cylinder—I did not think that the edge of a cylinder would produce such appearances upon the human body, until I performed the experiments.

The deceased's hair was gray; two or three gray hairs were found on the iron bar (*OB,* April 1864: pp. 477–78). Modern textbooks confirm Dr. Randall's experimental results.[3]

Specific marks were left on a body by certain objects, for example, by a rope used to bind a victim's wrists. On the breast of a woman who had been assaulted "there was an Impression of a Key, with all the Wards, stamp'd as plain, as if it had been made in Clay. I suppose she had the Key in her Bosom, and it was done by kneeling upon her"

3. See, for example, Adelson, 1974: p. 395.

(*OB*, Sept. 1733: p. 199). In another case a surgeon testified that "I examined a boot taken from one of the prisoners, and the heavy nails on the toe corresponded with the wound upon the policeman's forehead" (*OB*, Aug. 1876: p. 378).

Curiously enough, the significance of ecchymoses, or bruises, seems to have been infrequently recognized, although on one occasion a surgeon describing facial bruises remarked that "they were all recent except the black-eye, it was rather the remains of a black-eye, the bruise was of a greenish colour" (*OB*, June 1852: p. 233) His observation was significant in proving that the woman had been injured on two separate occasions.[4] Pathologists now recognize that bruises may be produced by trauma not only during life but also for a very short time after death and that a post-mortem bruise may be confused with livor, the discoloration that sometimes appears after death in dependent parts of the body as the blood settles by gravity. At the trial of James Greenacre and Sarah Gale for the notorious Edgware Road murder in 1837, it was established that the victim, a woman, had received a black eye before she was decapitated, since such an injury cannot be produced on a dead body: "A blow given half an hour after death would communicate lividity on the surface—I am speaking from experiment, from my own knowledge of the fact. . . . I am quite certain the appearance on the eye was the result of an injury inflicted during life, and not the results of *livor* after death. . . . I found the swelling in this case . . . as one of the symptoms of *ecchymosis* (*OB*, April 1837: pp. 895, 899–900).

In this same year Robert Christison published the results of his experiments on the effects of heavy blows delivered on the bodies, recently dead, of a dog and of four men and women. His conclusions about post-mortem contusions confirmed the above observation (1829b: pp. 236–50).

A particularly difficult problem at a post-mortem examination when multiple causes were found was to decide which one was primarily responsible for death. The answer could be crucial to the jury's decision in a homicide trial if it could be shown that there was more than one assailant. Such dilemmas were sometimes complicated by the differing opinions of medical witnesses for the defense and for the prosecution. In 1685 a woman was accused of striking or kicking an eleven-year-old girl in the abdomen; such an injury, said a surgeon,

4. The hue of a bruise changes over a period of days from purple to brown to green to yellow.

would be fatal. The accused woman claimed the girl died from "a Natural Disease," she being ill, "all of which was corroborated by another Chirurgeon that searched [examined] the Deceased." The court record does not enlighten us further (*OB,* July 1685: p. 3).

Two men had a fistfight for a wager. One of them died four days later; he had a history of gravel and urinary obstruction. A post-mortem examination disclosed abdominal bleeding and rupture of the intestine and urinary bladder. "*Q.* . . . you have no doubt that his death proceeded from the laceration of the intestines and the rupture of the bladder—*A.* Exactly so." But, the surgeon added, the bladder was diseased, and there were signs of "great inflammation on the surface of his bowels," which had resulted in adhesions. The liver and omentum were also adherent. "I consider the cause of his death to have been from a violent exertion, tearing away these adhesions; in this diseased state even if he had stumbled and endeavoured to recover himself, he might have done that mischief" (*OB,* May 1811: pp. 261–62).

During the cholera epidemic of 1832, an intoxicated woman succumbed after a fight and beating. No clear-cut marks of violence were discovered. Four surgeons expressed in court their opinion that she had died "of the prevailing epidemic cholera morbus" (*OB,* May 1832: pp. 532–34).

THE FÜHRHOP MURDER

Expert testimony presented at a murder trial in January 1865 illustrates contemporary forensic medical thinking. Ferdinand Edward Karl Kohl and Theodore Christian Führhop, two young Germans, were close friends and shared the same rooming house in East London. Kohl had complained that he wanted to return to Germany but lacked the money. Führhop had saved just enough to make a trip to New York and was ready to depart on Thursday, 3 November 1864. On the morning of that day the two young men went walking on the reedy bank of the Thames at Plaistow Marshes. About 1 P.M. Kohl returned alone, his clothes muddy. He reported that he and his friend had become separated in the Commercial Road. Kohl went out a second time, coming back about five; "he looked very bad when he came home then—his face looked pale, and his eyes sunk in his head." To a neighbor in the rooming house he returned a borrowed "chopper," a hatchet-like instrument. Kohl said he had put red paint on its top because the handle was loose. Later it developed that this handle was a replacement.

On Tuesday, 8 November, an apprentice hunting birds in Plaistow Marshes discovered the headless body of a man among the reeds. A police sergeant later testified that

> the body was lying on its back. . . . I observed the condition of the neck where the head had been severed from the body—there was a dent in the earth, apparently where the back of the head had been—small pieces of bone were lying by the neck, and a small portion of brain—the flesh had been eaten all round the bone, apparently by rats. . . . forty-five feet from where it was found I saw a quantity of blood, mixed with water, in a ditch. . . . about the same distance from where I found the blood I found this handle (*producing it*)—it is the handle of a hammer or hatchet.

On Sunday the thirteenth a knife was found twenty-two feet from the body. The missing head, partly buried, was located. A surgeon gave it as his opinion that "the cervical vertebrae had been severed as if by a chopper or some sharp instrument."

It was estimated that death had occurred four or five days before 8 November. Later, several head injuries, including fractures, were discovered. Some of the wounds had been produced by a blunt, some by a sharp instrument. The surgeon felt that both kinds could have been inflicted with the chopper. Asked whether decapitation had been carried out at the time of the murder or later, he expressed the opinion that it was "after the body was cold. . . . there was no muscular contractivity; the skin did not contract or the muscles either, which would be the case if cut off warm; it would be at least some hours after."

Testimony was heard from Dr. Henry Letheby (1816–76), a physician, analytical chemist, and professor of chemistry. For some time he was also food analyst and Medical Officer of Health for the City of London. He had, he stated, examined the chopper, and had determined that the paint had been applied after the new handle was inserted in the hatchet. On the edge of the weapon he had found

> a small quantity of brownish matter, which I removed and submitted to examination under the microscope. . . . I found some fibres of cotton and also some fibres of wool. . . . those fibres were bound together with a brownish matter, mixed with rust or iron; the nature of that brownish matter I could not determine. . . . I also found there some of the epithelium or surface skin of the human body; it was altogether mixed with this clot.
>
> COURT. Q. Can you distinguish the scales of the epithelium of the

human body from any other? *A.* Yes, the epithelium of the human body is very marked—I ascertained this to be human skin, I have no doubt about it.

On the basis of microscopic examination Letheby was not able to say whether the blood on the prisoner's coat was human; "it had all the characteristics of human blood—the blood of many other animals is like human blood—it was not the blood of a reptile, or of a bird, or of a fish."[5] He was convinced that the blood had clotted on the cloth shortly after leaving the body, since "blood immediately removed from the living animal coagulates by a spontaneous process—the coagulation had gone upon the cloth—the microscope does not discover albumen—the coagulation was fibrinous, not albuminous—the living coagulation is by fibrine, not albumen." A piece of the blood-stained cloth was then soaked in a few drops of water, yielding a colored solution; the latter could not be bleached with chlorine, "which will bleach almost any other colour" except that of blood.

The man who discovered the clasp knife in the reed bed "saw that it looked clean, and put it in my pocket—when I got home my wife made a remark that there were some hairs sticking out at the back of the spring." She added, "I saw two hairs sticking out. . . . it was very light hair—I should call it a very light brown." The knife was identified as having belonged to Kohl's wife, and the prisoner had been seen to use it. The clothes on the body were recognized as having been worn by Führhop.

The jury found Kohl guilty and he was sentenced to death (*OB,* Jan. 1865: pp. 161–80). It was not difficult for the forensic pathologist to relate the wounds on the body to chopper and knife, but full identification of the blood was rarely achieved in the days before the science of serology was established. Letheby did the best he could. The murderer had been remarkably careless. After killing Führhop with repeated chopper blows to the head, he managed with difficulty to decapitate the body, presumably to prevent its identification. He then transported the corpse forty-five feet from the gory scene. The handle of the chopper by now was loose and blood-stained; Kohl fitted a new handle and applied red paint, allegedly to tighten the handle but actually, it can be assumed, to cover blood on the head of the chopper. Then Kohl decided not to return the borrowed tool and threw it and the knife in different directions into the reeds. By this time his clothes

5. Fish, amphibians, reptiles, and some birds have nucleated red cells; man and most other mammals do not.

were spotted with paint and blood. He had not buried the head deep enough and rats exposed it. The clothes on the corpse were identified as those of Führhop.

CRUENTATION AND POST-MORTEM HEMORRHAGE

At least as early as the Middle Ages, it was believed that the corpse of a murdered man would bleed again if his killer drew near and touched the fatal wound. This flowing of blood was cruentation,[6] "the ordeal of the bier" (Cumston, 1912; Brittain, 1965). Shakespeare mentioned it in *Richard III,*

> O, gentlemen, see, see! dead Henry's wounds
> Open their congeal'd mouths and bleed afresh (1.2.55–56)

as did another Elizabethan, Michael Drayton (1932: 2, p. 333). King James I, enumerating tests for the detection of evildoers, included cruentation, "for as in a secret murther, if the deade carcase be at any time thereafter handled by the murtherer, it wil gush out of bloud, as if the blud wer crying to the heaven for revenge of the murtherer, God having appoynted that secret super-naturall signe, for tryall of that secrete vnnaturall crime" (James I, 1924: pp. 80–81).

In 1658 a Major Strangeways was accused of murdering his brother-in-law, John Fussel, by shooting him with a carbine. At the inquest, Strangeways was obliged to grasp the hand of the corpse and also to touch the wound. But the body did not bleed. Though the superstitious observers would have seen a flow of blood as evidence of Strangeway's guilt, with a strange inconsistency they refused to regard the absence of bleeding as an indication of innocence.

At his trial in the Old Bailey, the major refused to plead when he was charged with murder. Under the law, if an individual arraigned for a felony would not plead, he could not be found guilty, and thus his goods and chattels could not become forfeit to the Crown. Strangeways did not conceal his desire to preserve his lands for his heir, nor did he waver when duly warned that if he did not plead he would be sentenced to *peine forte et dure,* slow death by being crushed by heavy weights, a form of torture devised to force any prisoner to answer to his indictment. Unyielding, he died in the Press Yard at Newgate (Unhappy marksman, 1659).

6. From *cruentatus,* "bloody," "blood-stained."

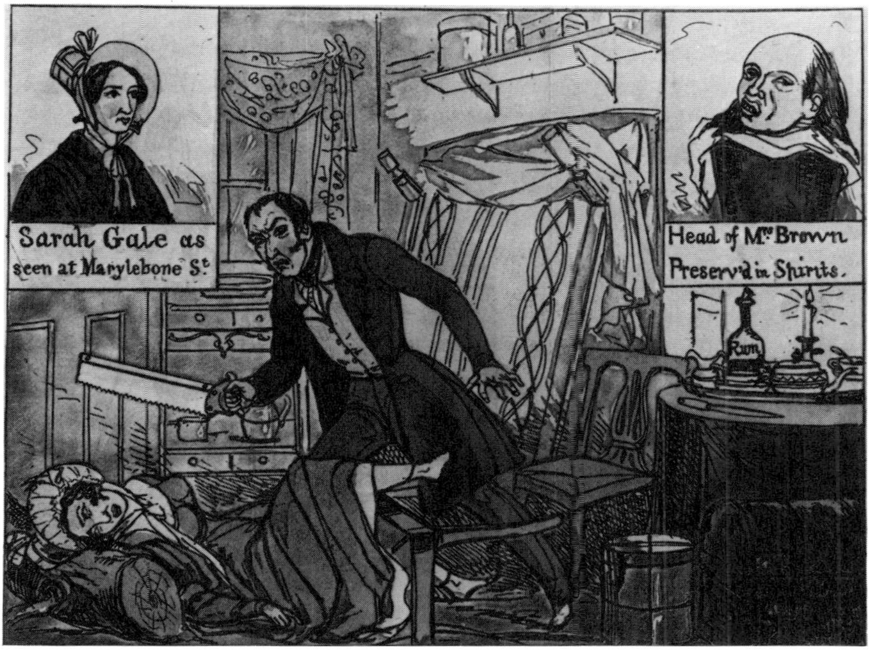
Sarah Gale as
seen at Marylebone St.
Head of Mrs Brown
Preserv'd in Spirits.
Rum

Murder of Hannah Brown by James Greenacre and Sarah Gale

Sir Walter Scott was much interested in cruentation, particularly in connection with the trial in 1688 in Edinburgh of Philip Stansfield for the murder of his father. The son had arranged for the body to be buried quickly, but foul play was suspected and the corpse was exhumed. Two surgeons performed an autopsy of sorts, then the remains were carefully washed and the relatives were requested to help to lift the body into its coffin. As the son raised his father's head, the bystanders saw blood appear through a linen wrapping around the neck. Philip dropped the corpse, staggered back in horror, and cried out, "Lord have mercy upon me!" When he was tried for murder, his counsel[7] dismissed as superstition any belief in the significance of the bleeding, but the prosecution made the most of the incident, failing at the same time, however, to mention that the autopsy report also described a cervical dislocation, quite possibly the real cause of death. Philip Stansfield was found guilty.[8] Popular belief in cruentation as a

7. At this time Scottish law permitted counsel for the defense in a felony trial.
8. Glaister, 1897; Davison, 1964; Brittain, 1965.

proof of guilt persisted into the nineteenth century; according to Chaillé, the practice survived as a legal expedient in New York as late as 1824 (1949: p. 401f).

Although not provoked by the touch of a murderer, post-mortem bleeding is possible. At the murder trial of Greenacre and Gale in 1837, forensic scientists were unable to agree on the circumstances permitting bleeding after death. Guy, a contemporary writer on forensic medicine, believed that "copious hemorrhage will be a reason for supposing a wound to have been inflicted during life, and the entire absence of it . . . an equally strong reason for attributing death to some other cause. Lacerated wounds, however, may bleed very little during life, and a large severed vein may bleed extensively after death" (1845: p. 450). His opinion is probably closest to the modern viewpoint.

In summary, forensic medical understanding of the significance of wounds evolved slowly. If a wounded man died, cause and effect seemed obvious and that was the end of the matter. When, exceptionally, the body was "opened," an appropriate term for a usually perfunctory procedure, examination of the organs was brief. The surgeon looked only for what he expected to see. How often was death ascribed to a visible wound when the victim had in fact died of an unrecognized skull fracture or of hidden hemorrhage from a lung pierced by a broken rib? How many times would a careful autopsy have disclosed evidence that a fatal accident had occurred subsequent to the assault or that there had been a second assailant? Why did prosecutor, judge, or jury not press for such crucial information? We can only conclude that its importance too often escaped all concerned. All, that is, except the prisoner in the dock.

III

Injuries to the Central Nervous System

THE CENTRAL NERVOUS SYSTEM IS RATHER WELL PROTECTED BY MUScles, ligaments, membranes, bones, and fluid, but when these defenses are penetrated, or when the system is shaken with sufficient violence, the trauma to the remarkably delicate brain and spinal cord can be disastrous. The correct interpretation of the causation of such injuries was sometimes a difficult and intricate problem for the autopsy surgeon, but the life and liberty of an accused person repeatedly depended on his perception, thoroughness, experience, and knowledge.

SINGLE INJURY BY BLUNT OBJECT

It is well known that, of all parts of the body, the head is particularly vulnerable to violent contact with blunt objects (Adelson, 1974: p. 397). A frequent result of such injury was the rupture of one of the meningeal or cerebral blood vessels or of the dural sinuses, all of which lie between the brain and the inner surface of the skull. Percivall Pott, the distinguished London surgeon, testified regarding such injuries.[1] The autopsy followed a death from skull fracture resulting from

1. Pott (1714–88), a teacher of John Hunter, wrote classic accounts of a variety of leg fracture and of tuberculosis of the spine. He was the author of the first description of congenital hernia, of an important work on head injuries (1773), and of a paper on the frequency of scrotal cancer in chimney sweeps, early recognition of a malignant tumor of occupational origin. For expert testimony by Pott at another trial see Forbes, 1975.

a blow with a stick:

> I view'd the Body externally, and found two Bruises, one above the Right-ear, and the other over the Right-eye. There was a large Fracture in the Skull. . . . The [top of the] Skull being remov'd, I found 8 ounces of extravasated Blood, part between the first Skin [dura] and the skull, another part between the first Skin and the Second, and the rest in the two lateral Ventricles of the Brain. The Skull being broke in, was the Occasion of her Death. (*OB,* Mar. 1734: p. 88)

Bleeding from a ruptured venous sinus of the dura mater usually resulted from ante-mortem trauma. However, as a careful witness pointed out in 1863, tearing of the sinus could also occur during lifting of the calvaria, or top of the skull, at autopsy. A surgeon made a post-mortem examination less than three hours after a man died during a prize fight. The skull was not fractured. Upon

> removing the skull-cap I found a large coagulum of congested blood on both hemispheres of the brain, which was congested—all the other organs were perfectly healthy—I attribute death to the effusion of blood on the brain, which could be caused by a blow at a prize fight. . . . the [superior] longitudinal *sinus* was ruptured in two places—I could not say whether that was produced before death or after—great force is required in removing the skull-cap—this clot could not have been caused by the removal of the skull-cap. (*OB,* May 1873: pp. 160–66)

This appears to have been an acute subdural hematoma, perhaps resulting from rupture of the sinus. But the surgeon could not be sure whether the rupture occurred during the prize fight or later, during the post-mortem examination.

Some fatal head injuries from blows were described as "concussion of the brain," a term in conflict with the modern viewpoint, which holds that concussion rarely causes death (J. G. Greenfield, 1958: p. 408; Bannister, 1978: p. 248). Concussion was reported in Old Bailey testimony in 1810. A man was knocked down repeatedly in a fight. The victim, unconscious and with symptoms allegedly denoting concussion, succumbed forty-three hours after he was seen by a surgeon. The latter made an autopsy and observed what would now be termed an acute subdural hemorrhage with compression of the brain: "Q. If this rupture had taken place from any act during the fight, could the person have walked away from the place after the fight, in the manner as described, without any symptoms of concussion of the brain?—A. I believe not" (*OB,* April 1810: p. 174). The surgeon's perhaps incorrect answer to the query very likely explains why the prisoner was found not guilty.

PUNCTURE WOUNDS

Penetration of the skull by a pointed object seems to have been a relatively uncommon type of injury. In an early case, a young man was struck with a blunt weapon or punched on the *left* side of his head. He fell, bled heavily from the nose, soon collapsed, and died. A small wound, about the size that would be made by a lancet, was discovered just above his *right* ear. At autopsy the careful and perceptive surgeon

> found a Perforation thro' the Skull, triangular, and about the Bigness of the End of *this* Probe, and a great Quantity of coagulated Blood between the two Membranes of the Brain. The Perforation thro' the Skull answered directly to the Wound in the Flesh, above the Ear. I take the Perforation to have been made by a Nail. . . . I apprehend that from the blow given on the opposite Side of the Head, he might fall upon something Sharp, which gave him that Wound; and there was a Blackness [bruise] on the opposite side of the Head. (*OB*, Dec. 1736: pp. 37–38)

We can now surmise that the hemorrhage might also have been due to a basal skull fracture. Directly or indirectly, the blow to the head resulted in death.

MULTIPLE INJURIES

John Hunter appeared as an expert witness on several occasions.[2] In 1784 a London constable, Nicholas Casson, was struck on the left side of the head with a bludgeon, knocked to the street, and kicked. He lived only a few hours. At the trial of four men accused of Casson's murder, Hunter first spoke of finding broken ribs at the autopsy:

> I next examined the head. . . . I observed extravasated blood where a blow most probably had been received. When the skull was removed we observed more blood to issue than is common; at the first membrane of the skull [dura mater], we found opposite to the extravasated blood, a considerable quantity of coagulated blood laying between the two membranes of the brain. We examined the scull on the inside, and *opposite* to that from where the first extravasated blood had appeared, there was found several fractures [italics added].
>
> *Court.* Were those [fractures] the occasions of his death?—No,

2. Hunter, younger brother of William and Britain's leading medical scientist of the eighteenth century, was renowned for his investigations in anatomy, surgery, and experimental biology. Less well known but also important were his contributions as a forensic pathologist.

> those were the appearances of it; the extravasated blood found on the right side, opposite to where the blow was given, was the cause of his death.

Thus, after Casson was knocked down by a blow from a bludgeon on the left side of the head, the right side of his skull was fractured, either by impact with the pavement, by a second blow from a club, or by a kick. If Hunter was correct in believing that Casson died because of brain damage associated with the skull fracture on the right, then the initial blow on the left, observed by witnesses, would only have contributed to his death, and the guilt of his first assailant would have been somewhat less.

The court next asked Hunter, "What do you suppose the [first] blow was given with?" His answer is instructive:

> I should suppose it was given by a blunt instrument. A sharp heavy instrument, such as a rod of iron, will make a very considerable external appearance [lesion], perhaps greater than an internal one, but an instrument of a considerable size, and with considerable velocity, may make no external appearance, because it covers so large a surface, but it may give the head such a shock, such a quick velocity, as to produce extravasation. (*OB,* June 1784: p. 668; Forbes, 1980)

The jury decided that the accused men were innocent. John Hunter's comments on cranial trauma here, and also in his *Lectures on the Principles of Surgery,* published posthumously (1839: pp. 256–63), are noteworthy for his clear understanding of the mechanics of head injury, an understanding seldom reflected in the forensic medical testimony of other surgeons, even well into the nineteenth century.

An intoxicated man, George Reeves, fell out of his donkey cart onto the pavement, began scuffling with a bystander, and was struck on the head with a brush. Soon after, Reeves became unconscious, and died two days later. At the post-mortem examination, an epidural hemorrhage—bleeding between the outer membrane and the inside of the skull—resulting from rupture of a small artery was found. In the opinion of the surgeon, "A heavy fall from the cart might cause such an injury, but then he would have had symptoms of unconsciousness at the time; I think the rupture took place at the second assault, I believe he was unconscious after that" (*OB,* Oct. 1878: pp. 694–95).

The medical witness was incorrectly convinced that unconsciousness always rapidly follows a large cerebral hemorrhage. When there were two cranial insults separated by an interval of several minutes or hours, and when evidence of fatal intracranial bleeding was found at autopsy, the medical man was led to believe that the *second* injury was responsible for death. Such a determination could be decisive in the jury's decision in a homicide trial. But it had actually been known for almost half a century that unconsciousness does not necessarily follow immediately after a head injury. Alfred Swaine Taylor wrote in 1836:

> It must be remembered, that in cases of injuries to the head proving fatal by extravasation of blood on the brain, an individual may recover from the first effects of the violence, and apparently be going on well, when he will suddenly become worse and die. Extravasation takes place slowly at first . . . but after a shorter or longer period, the haemorrhage will recur and destroy life by producing compression. . . . How many hours or days, after an accident, are required in order that such an increased effusion should take place, it is impossible to say; but in severe cases, fatal extravasation is observed to follow the injury within a very short time. (pp. 417, 418)

CONTRECOUP

Contrecoup injuries to intracranial blood vessels and cerebral tissues occur as follows.[3] When the unsupported head is struck powerfully on one side, in front, or in back, the skull is moved violently. Due to the inertia of the brain, it in turn is deformed against the moving skull. Correspondingly, that portion of the brain on the opposite side of the head moves abruptly *away* from the skull. This last shift may result in tearing of the arachnoid and pia mater, rupture of fine trabeculae and meningeal and cerebral vessels, and damage to brain tissue itself, all in the contrecoup area. Contrecoup injuries to the cranial contents may also result when the rapidly moving head is stopped abruptly, as in a fall to the pavement. By a different mechanism, a contrecoup fracture of the skull may occur on the side opposite the external point of impact.[4]

Post-mortem examination of a man who had been punched in the head, knocked down, and kicked in the face showed bruises and lacerations of the nose and right eyebrow. Opening the skull revealed hemorrhage at the base of the brain and within the ventricles; "it was a case of *contre coup*—it was pressing on the *medulla oblongata*" (*OB*, Nov. 1871: pp. 35–36). In this instance the impact was delivered high

3. The French term *contrecoup* was used in English as early as 1830, in Samuel Cooper's *The First Lines of the Practice of Surgery*.

4. Gonzales et al., 1937: p. 157; J. G. Greenfield, 1958: pp. 409–19; Adelson, 1974: pp. 400, 428.

on the front of the head and the contrecoup injury was low in the back of the cranial cavity.

APOPLEXY

Ficarra (1977, p. 4) reminds us that until the investigations of Johann Jacob Wepfer in the middle of the seventeenth century, it was usually believed that apoplexy resulted from external cranial injury. The latter's *Observationes anatomicae, ex cadaveribus eorum, quos sustulit apoplexia* (Anatomical observations on the bodies of those who succumbed to apoplexy), published in 1658, declared, in effect, that apoplexy was caused by interference with the circulation of the brain, including obstruction of the carotid or vertebral arteries or jugular veins.[5] Wepfer concluded that a major cranial hemorrhage could also cause apoplexy. Such an effusion would result from opening of cerebral vascular anastomoses or from rupture, laceration, or erosion of the cerebral vessels (Donley, 1909).

A man choked his wife. She was cared for by a barber surgeon—"I only practice bleeding, and operations on the teeth"—who bled her freely and felt the woman was improved, but she died about twelve hours after being attacked. A surgeon testified at the inquest that the autopsy did not reveal the cause of death, "upon which the [coroner's] jury adjourned, that we might make a further enquiry. I was called upon again, this day fortnight, and another surgeon was sent for, and upon opening the head . . . we found" an intracranial hemorrhage, caused by choking and resulting in apoplexy. John Hunter, the second surgeon at the autopsy, concurred (*OB,* May 1753: pp. 133–34: Forbes, 1980). Note the interval of two weeks between the first and second autopsies and the commendable persistence of the coroner's jury.

Dunglison in his textbook warned that

> a person may be seized with apoplexy in a place where there are hard or sharp objects on which he falls, and extensive wounds, with loss of blood, may be the consequence—dissection will shew that death has

5. Wepfer (1620–95), a brilliant Swiss medical man and comparative anatomist, also made careful studies on the actions of poisons. Appointed physician to his native city of Schaffhausen, he was permitted to perform post-mortem examinations. Wepfer's detailed description of what came to be called the circle of Willis antedated by several years Thomas Willis's description (1664) of the same vessels. Willis's account does not mention Wepfer's report.

> not been the consequence of external violence,—or, he may fall in the apoplectic state into water and be taken out dead—in such a case the signs of apoplexy will probably be manifest. . . . A person again may fall from a height in an apoplectic fit and fracture his skull. (1827: p. 13)

SUNSTROKE

Conflicting expert testimony was involved in a manslaughter trial in which the central issue was whether the death of a ten-year-old boy was due to a blow or to sunstroke. The victim, struck on the top of his head by the closed fist of his schoolmaster, seemed dazed, complained of a severe headache, had a rapid pulse, and vomited repeatedly. These symptoms continued for several days; he was unable to urinate, staggered when he walked, and complained of photophobia. The boy became progressively more ill, and died twenty days after he was injured. During all this time the weather had been exceptionally warm. The autopsy surgeon found inflammation and thickening of the meninges under the top of the skull and ascribed the symptoms and pathology to the blow. A second surgeon, who claimed much experience with sunstroke cases in India and China, saw the boy before death and found no indication of external violence. He swore that death was due to sunstroke. The prisoner was found not guilty (*OB,* Nov. 1868: pp. 34–36).

OTHER PATHOLOGY

A few homicide trials involved deaths due to lesions of the brain that were apparently unrelated to recent violence. Dr. John Reid (1841) reported the case of a man accidentally struck on the side of the head in the fall of a small bale of cotton. He collapsed, later became delirious, and died a week after he was injured. Autopsy revealed that the ventricles of the brain were distended with water. Later it was discovered that he had suffered "a severe injury on the head" *eighteen months* previously. Reid concluded that the cerebral damage was the result of the original trauma. This may have been a case of communicating hydrocephalus secondary to subarachnoid hemorrhage incurred at the time of the original injury.

Rather large numbers both of accused persons and of their alleged victims were described in court, often euphemistically, as having been under the influence of alcohol. Not only did intoxication sometimes play a role in the events leading to a homicide but, in the opinion of expert witnesses, inebriation or its long-term effects could be a contributing cause of death. Nineteenth-century medical men recognized, incidentally, that delirium tremens is not always associated with alcholism. An adult male who was repeatedly punched about the head became delirious three days later. The patient succumbed, said his surgeon, "of exhaustion, of *delirium tremens,* which I attribute to the shock that the system had received from the injuries on the side of the face, at the time of the affray." There was no skull fracture (*OB,* Oct. 1846: pp. 874–77).

Alfred Swaine Taylor cautiously observed in 1836 that

> a [medical] witness may be asked whether he can distinguish between the effects of *concussion* and *intoxication*. The history of the individual will sometimes suffice to establish a distinction, but this cannot always be obtained. It is commonly said that the odour of the breath will detect intoxication; but it is obvious that a man may meet with concussion after having drunk liquor insufficient to cause intoxication, or concussion may take place while he is intoxicated. . . . The examiner should weigh all the circumstances, and if there be one cause of the symptoms more *probable* than another, let him adopt it:—if not, let him give the benefit of the doubt to the accused party. It is better than ten guilty men should escape, than that one, who is innocent, should suffer! (p. 417)

SPINAL CORD INJURY

Fatal injury to the brain was reported much more frequently in expert testimony than was trauma to the spinal cord, but a few instances of the latter were described. The details of one such case were presented in 1831 at the trial of John Bishop, Thomas Williams, and James May for the murder of Carlo Ferrari, the "Italian boy," as he came to be called in the press. The crime was committed in order to obtain a body for sale to the anatomists.

The study of human anatomy, an indispensable part of medical training, required a continuing supply of cadavers. Under English law, only the bodies of executed felons could properly be made available for dissection. With the rapid increase in numbers of medical students in London in the second half of the eighteenth century, the supply of legally released cadavers became quite inadequate. Teachers of anatomy were faced with the choice of depriving medical students of an essential part of their training or using illegal sources for bodies. As a result, teachers, their assistants, and their students—and later professional "resurrection men"—turned to grave-robbing. The sale of stolen cadavers became a lucrative and well-organized activity. The violation of graves was often discovered, and public outrage grew with each fresh scandal, but grave-robbing continued for many years.

Continental countries had for centuries met the need for cadavers for dissection by the simple expedient of legally releasing unclaimed bodies to the schools of anatomy. Parliamentary reform of British laws to make possible a similar procedure was repeatedly urged, and the trial in Edinburgh in 1828 of the notorious Burke and Hare, who had turned to murder to procure bodies, particularly stimulated the clamor for change. Further shocking disclosures were made three years later when Bishop and his associates were brought to justice in London for a similar offense. As a result, in 1832 Parliament passed the Warburton Anatomy Act, instituting at last the means for providing a sufficient legal supply of bodies.

But to return to the trial at the Old Bailey. A witness described what occurred when Bishop and May arrived at the medical school to negotiate a sale:

> WILLIAM HILL. I am porter at the dissecting-room at King's college, Somerset-house.[6] On Saturday, the 5th of November, about a quarter to twelve o'clock, the bell of the dissecting-room rang: I answered it, and found Bishop and May at the door—I knew them before; May asked if I wanted anything—I said not particularly, and asked what he had got; he said a male subject; I asked him what size—he said it was a boy about fourteen years of age: I asked the price: he said twelve guineas—I said I could not think of giving that price for it; we did not care much about it, for we did not particularly want it, but if he would wait I would see Mr. Partridge, who is the demonstrator of anatomy.

Partridge, Hill, and the malefactors bargained for a while, finally agreeing on a price of nine guineas. About 2:15 P.M. May, Bishop, and two confederates returned with a burden.

> all four persons stood around the hamper. . . . May and Bishop carried the hamper through into the other room, they opened it between them, and in it was a sack, containing the body in question. . . . both

6. King's College, founded in 1829, occupied the east wing of Somerset House in the Strand.

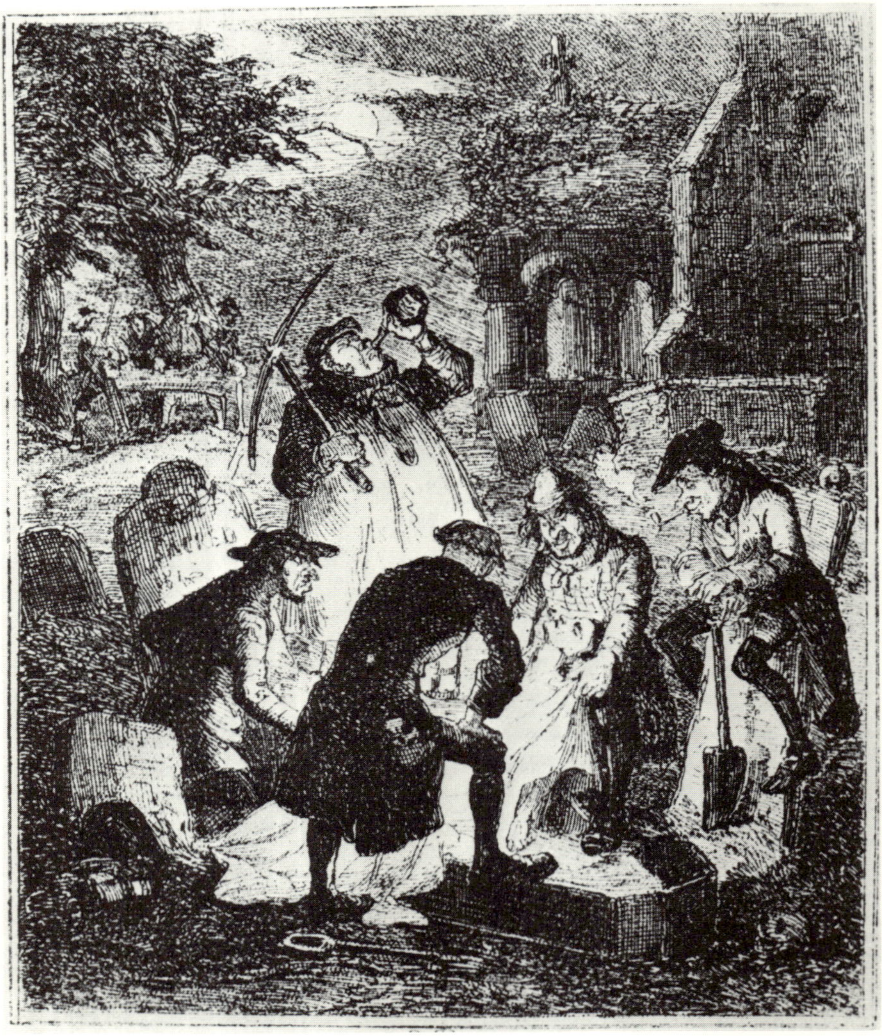

The Resurrectionists

May and Bishop observed that we could not have a fresher, or that it was a very good, one—I said Yes, it was certainly fresh . . . and made some remarks upon it to myself, in consequence of which I went to Mr. Partridge; I asked the prisoners what the body had died with; they said they did not know, it was no business of mine or theirs. . . . I know the body had not been laid out in a coffin, for there was no saw-dust about the head.

Bishop, ever greedy, found a moment alone with the porter to make a private deal. Said the latter, "as I left the room the body was in, Bishop said that when I paid them I was to give him only eight guineas in the presence of Williams [another confederate], and to give him the other guinea, and he would give me half a crown."

Hill and Partridge, the demonstrator in anatomy, by now more than a little suspicious that death had not been due to natural causes, quietly sent for the police, then returned to where May and Bishop were waiting. Partridge delayed the men on a pretext until the constables arrived and took them into custody.

Partridge testified as to his suspicions when he was shown the body: "I observed the swollen state of the face, the blood-shot eyes, the freshness of the body, the rigidity of the limbs,[7] and a cut over the left temple; the lips were swollen." The next day Partridge and others conducted a post-mortem examination:

> There was a wound on the temple, which did not injure the bone—that was the only appearance of external injury; on the scull, beneath the scalp or bone there was some blood effused; on opening the body the whole contents of the abdomen and chest were found to be in a healthy condition. . . . [the brain] was perfectly healthy, as well as the spinal part; in cutting down to remove the bone which conceals the spinal part at the back of the neck, we found a quantity of coagulated blood within the muscles, and on removing the back part of the bony [vertebral] canal, some coagulated blood was found laying in the cavity opposite the blood found in the muscles of the neck. . . . the spinal marrow appeared perfectly healthy. . . . I think these internal marks of violence were sufficient to produce death. . . .
>
> *Q*. Must those appearances have been produced by some cause inflicted on the back of the neck? *A*. I believe so; I think a blow from a stick on the back of the neck would have caused those appearances. . . . I am not aware that the appearances on the spinal cord would be found in persons dying a natural death.

A second surgeon confirmed these observations, adding that neither apoplexy nor a blow on top of the head would have produced the pathological conditions described. This witness also disclosed that the victim's teeth had been extracted post-mortem, with damage to the gums and jaws.

Another witness, a waiter in a public house, stated that on the evening before May and Bishop were arrested, the former "went to

7. Rigor mortis usually sets in six to twelve hours after death, persists for about twelve hours, and disappears after another twelve hours or more. Partridge meant that the body had not long been dead.

the bar with something in a silk handkerchief, which afterwards turned out to be teeth, for I saw him pour water on the silk handkerchief and rub the teeth in his hand—he afterwards opened the handkerchief, so that I could see they were human teeth; I remarked to May that they appeared to be young ones, and were worth a few shillings—he said they were worth *2l.* to him." The transplantation of teeth was not unusual in the eighteenth and part of the nineteenth century, generating demand for human teeth in good condition, for which high prices were paid (Hunter, 1778: *2,* 94–112; Bremner, 1954: p. 102).

A porter and his assistant at Guy's Hospital and the "procurator [of bodies] at Mr. Grainger's anatomical theatre" all testified that Bishop and May had tried to sell them the body of a boy aged about fourteen (*OB,* Dec. 1831: pp. 24–33).

Bishop, May, and Williams were found guilty and were sentenced to death. The 5 December 1831 issue of *The Gentleman's Magazine* noted their execution at the Old Bailey, "when a number of persons were severely injured, owing to the presence of the vast crowd. May was respited" (1831: 101, 461,643).

Clearly the understanding of head injuries in the eighteenth century presented many problems to the medical man. Aside from John Hunter and Percivall Pott, few British surgeons displayed any real grasp of the mechanics and pathology of cranial trauma. Animal experiments in this field were rare, and the surgeon turned too often to conjecture as he tried to understand cause and effect. When multiple causes of death were suspected, temporal factors, sometimes crucially important in determining the guilt or innocence of the accused, were poorly understood. In addition, the frequent failure to perform a thorough post-mortem examination on occasion almost certainly masked significant noncranial lesions.

By the middle of the nineteenth century, improved knowledge of the neuropathologic results of trauma was beginning to be manifested in forensic medical testimony. The contributions of the great Frenchman Paul Broca (1824–80) and others were laying a foundation which would eventually strengthen the surgeon's understanding of the central nervous system and result in the modern specialty of neurosurgery. More and better medicolegal autopsies helped to dispel some of the mystery that had obscured cranial trauma. But progress was slow, not least in the field of forensic medicine, where the dissemination and utilization of knowledge seems to have lagged well behind its discovery. And head injuries remained a leading cause of violent death.

IV

Asphyxia

When for some reason, sufficient oxygen does not reach the lungs and thus the blood, and carbon dioxide accumulates excessively in the blood instead of being discharged by expiration, coma ensues and may end in death. This condition is known as asphyxia. The fatal lack of oxygen may result from strangulation, smothering, and so on, or from inhalation of a mixture such as smoke containing little or no free oxygen. Adelson points out that certain asphyxiating homicidal and suicidal procedures, for example hanging, also cause compression of blood vessels in the neck, leading in turn to lethal interference with the circulation to the brain. Cervical pressure may in addition induce a fatal carotid sinus reflex (Adelson, 1974: pp. 522, 526–27).

SIMULATED HANGING

In the year 1514 one Richard Hunne was a respected citizen and merchant tailor of the City of London, "a man of good Substance, a fair Dealer, and also a good Catholick." Because the forensic medical aspects of this important case (History, 1725; Wunderli, 1982) seem to have been almost forgotten, it is recounted here in some detail. The story begins innocently enough. Hunne's infant was being cared for in the Parish of St. Mary Matfelon, later known as St. Mary Whitechapel, near the City. The baby died, and was buried by the parish. The parish clerk, who was also the parson, demanded the bearing sheet as his mortuary.[1] Hunne refused, on the grounds that the child had not owned the sheet and that the parson had no claim on it. The clergyman, quite without conscience, thereupon summoned the father to appear in the ecclesiastical court, setting in motion an increasingly ugly sequence of events:

> The Citizen well considering he was like to be born down there [in court], apply'd himself to Counsel learned in the Law for Advice, who instructed him to bring a Writ of *Praemunire*[2] against the Parson and all his Aiders, Counsellors, Proctors and Adherents.
>
> Now the Clergy in general taking Alarm at this Proceeding, and being apprehensive [that] if they should suffer their Brother to be cast [defeated] at the Suit of *Hunne,* a Door would thereby be open'd for others of the Laity to serve other Clergymen in the same manner, there were no endeavours wanting to bring Hunne within the Danger of their Ecclesiastical Laws, and at length they found a way to accuse him of Heresy, before Dr. *Richard Fitz-James,* then Bishop of *London,* who ordered him to be confined a Prisoner in the *Lollard Tower* at *St. Paul's*[3] and so close that none of his Friends should be allowed to come near him.

On 2 December 1514 the unfortunate Hunne was brought before Dr. Horsey, the Chancellor of the Bishop of London, to be examined on five charges of heresy. Hunne's answers are not recorded, but a signed partial admission of guilt is written under the list of his alleged sins. According to the chronicler, the handwriting of the admission might have been that of another person: "Hoc fuit Scriptum manu propria Richardi Hunne ut dicitur" ("this was written by the hand of Richard Hunne himself *as it was said*"), that is, by hearsay. The examination over, the prisoner was returned to the Lollards' Tower and put in the custody of John Spalding, the bell ringer.

On the morning of 4 December Hunne was found hanged in his prison cell. Earlier that day Spalding had departed,

> leaving the Keys of the Prison with one of his Fellows, to deliver them to the Sumner's Boy,[4] who was wont to carry Victuals and other

1. A bearing sheet was a cloth with which a baby was covered when it was baptized; a mortuary was a kind of ecclesiastical fee claimed by a minister on the death of a parishioner (Black, 1968: p. 1163).

2. A writ that could be used to prevent or repress papal encroachment and usurpation. It reflected the anticlerical sentiment of the period.

3. Speaking of the old St. Paul's Cathedral, Stow says, "At either corner of this west end . . . is a strong tower of stone, made for bell towers . . . [that] towards the south, is called the Lowlarde's tower, and hath been used as the bishop's prison, for such as were detected for opinions in religion, contrary to the faith of the church" (1970: p. 330).

4. A summoner was an official who ordered persons to appear in court, particularly an ecclesiastical court.

> Necessaries to the Prisoner, their Intention being this, That the Boy first finding *Hunne* dead, they, by his Account, might be thought free from all manner of Suspicion, which indeed at first succeeded according to their wishes. For the Boy, with two others of the Bishop's Sumners, going into the Prison to serve him as usual, and finding him hang'd with his Face to the Wall, they were frighted, and immediately ran to the Chancellor, then in the Church, with the horible News, who forthwith with some of his Colleagues going into the Prison, it was immediately given out that *Hunne* had in desperation hang'd himself. And so the Rumour passed currently at first, and the Murderers began to think themselves safe from all manner of Discovery.

Fortunately an inquest was opened, and the coroner and his jury set to work. Meanwhile, "the Bishop of London went to Work another way, and proceeded *ex officio,* as in Case of *Heresy* against the Deceased; imagining, as likely, that if he were once condemn'd of Heresy, the Inquest could do no less than find him guilty of Self-Murder [*felo de se,* suicide]." So the bishop collected thirteen additional heresies from the prologue of Hunne's English bible, now in the possession of this churchman. Both sets of heresies were read out publicly at St. Paul's the next Sunday, together with a solemn warning to all those who might share Hunne's alleged views.

> After this open Publication and Admonition, the Bishop examin'd divers of the Clergy and some Laymen, about the Contents of these Articles, and among others they had a Man and a Maid Servant of *Hunne*'s under Examination. They had liv'd with him a long while, but could not Charge him with any thing of moment worth Reprehension; nay, they could say nothing at all to the Articles [of heresy] chiefly objected against him. However, divers of the Priests charg'd him with the Guilt of one Article, some with another, and design'd to proceed speedily to a Sentence of Condemnation.

A public session of the ecclesiastical court was held, and the dead Richard Hunne was found guilty of multiple heresies:

> There were present in Court, besides the Bishop of *London,* those of *Durham* and *Lincoln,* with many Doctors both in Divinity and the Canon Law, so that what they did was look'd upon as an Act of the whole Clergy, and what was done by them was, to Sentence his dead Body to be burnt, and having deliver'd the same to the Secular Power, it was executed accordingly on the 20th of *December* 1514, in *Smithfield,*[5] sixteen Days after he had been barbarously murder'd. . . .
>
> This Proceeding produc'd more different Effects than what was really expected. For it was hop'd, that *Hunne* being found a Heretick, no body for the future would have stirr'd in his behalf. Whereas on the contrary, it occasion'd loud Clamours, the Man having liv'd in very

5. Market place and site of executions.

good Reputation amongst his Neighbours, so that from thence forward the City of *London* was never well affected to the *Popish* Clergy. . . .

There might be hopes indeed that all this Clamour would be over in time, and the thing forgot; what grated most for the present, was the Coroner's Inquest, who were extreamly diligent in their Duty. They were several times sent for before the Privy Council, and the King himself sometimes present; at other times they appear'd before the Chief Judges and Justices of the Kingdom, who observing how the Clergy interested themselves in the Affair, it was left wholly to the Inquest, who found Dr. *Horsey,* the Bishop of *London's* Chancellor, *Charles Joseph,* his Sumner, and *John Spalding,* the Bell-Ringer of *St. Paul's,* had committed the Murder upon the Body of Richard Hunne.

The Bishop of London, anxious to dispose of Hunne's corpse and thereby of incriminating evidence, had acted with some dispatch to arrange through the ecclesiastical court to have the sentence of burning carried out. But the bishop was not quick enough. The body had been discovered on 4 December. The Coroner of the City of London, William Barnwell, moved by zeal—a rather uncommon attribute of coroners in those days—and perhaps also by strong anticlerical sentiment, had held his inquest on 5 and 6 December in the Ward of Castle Baynard.[6] The coroner's inquisition, that is, the document reporting the findings of the inquest, is remarkable for perception and thoroughness. It relates how the coroner and his twenty-four jurymen had gone to the Lollards' Tower,

where we found the Body of the said *Hunne* hanging upon a Staple of Iron, in a Girdle of Silk, with fair Countenance, hair kemmed [combed], and his Bonnet right fitting upon his Head, with the Eyes and Mouth fair closed, without any Stirring, Gaping, or Frowning, also without any driveling or sparging [spattering] in any part of his Body. Whereupon by one Assent we all agreed to take down the body of the said *Hunne,* and as soon as we began to heave the Body it was loose, whereby by good Advisement we perceived, that the Girdle had no knot about the Staple, but it was double cast [doubled], and the Links of an Iron Chain, which did hang on the Iron Staple, were laid upon the same Girdle, whereby it did hang; also the knot of the Girdle that went about his Neck stood under his Left Ear, which caused his Head to lean towards his Right Shoulder: notwithstanding there came out of his Nostrils two small Streams of Blood, to the Quantity of four Drops; save only those four Drops of Blood, the Face, Chin, Doublet, Collar and Shirt of the said *Hunne,* was clear from any

6. The location of St. Paul's Cathedral. It was customary to hold an inquest in the ward in which the death under investigation had occurred.

> Blood: Also we find, that both the Skin of his Neck and Throat beneath the Girdle of Silk, was freat [fretted, excoriated] and fallen away with that thing [with] which the Murderers had broken his Neck withal: Also the Hands of the said *Hunne* were wrung in the Wrists whereby we perceived that his hands had been bound. Moreover, we find that within the said Prison was no means whereby any Man might hang himself, but only a Stool, which Stool stood upon a Bolster of a Bed, so tickled [precariously balanced], that any Man or Beast might not touch it so little but it was ready to fall; whereby we perceived that it was not possible that *Hunne* might hang himself, the Stool so standing. Also all the Girdle from the Staple to his Neck was too little for his Head to come out thereat. Also it was not possible that the soft Silken Girdle could break his Neck, or Skin beneath the Girdle. Also we find in a Corner somewhat beyond the Place where he did hang, a great Parcel of Blood. Also we find upon the Left side of *Hunne*'s Jacket, from the Breast downwards, two great Streams of Blood. Also within the Flap of the Left side of his Jacket, we find a Cluster of Blood, and the Jacket folden down thereupon; which thing the said *Hunne* could never fold nor do after he was hang'd. Whereby it appeareth plainly to us all, that the Neck of *Hunne* was broken, and the great Plenty of Blood was shed before he was hang'd. Wherefore all we find by God and all our Consciences, that *Richard Hunne* was murder'd. Also we acquit the said *Richard Hunne* of his own Death.

Now consider the findings thus far. Remember that public hangings were common in the sixteenth century and that onlookers were familiar with the appearance of a corpse after execution. At that time, a judicial hanging resulted in death by asphyxia, the "drop" not being far enough to produce a cervical fracture. The coroner's jurymen would have been familiar with the characteristic bluish or dusky hue of the skin (cyanosis), protrusion of the tongue, and signs of a terminal struggle observed in a hanged man or woman.

But the body in the Lollards' Tower had "a fair countenance," the hair was combed, the bonnet was not disarranged, "his Eyes and Mouth fair closed, without any Stirring, Gaping, or Frowning." The silk girdle, intended to look like a noose, was *not* knotted to the iron staple from which the corpse was suspended. It appears that the supporting iron chain encircled the neck *outside* the girdle. After the girdle was tied, there was not enough slack for the head to have been inserted into the loop of cloth.

The neck, said the inquisition, had been broken with a "thing" by the murderers. This lethal object had excoriated the skin of the throat; such abrasions could not have been produced by the soft material of the girdle. After suspension of the body, the skin of the neck was protected from scraping by the chain because of the underlying fabric of the girdle. Therefore, the neck was broken *before* suspension of the body.

The wrists showed signs of having been bound. The rope or cord presumably had been removed to make suicide look plausible.

It is implied but not stated that the feet of the suspended corpse were not touching the floor and that a suicidal Hunne would have had to stand on and step off a stool or similar object. But the only stool was precariously balanced some distance away on the bolster of a bed, "whereby we perceived that it was not possible that *Hunne* might hang himself, the Stool so standing."

The inquisition says that blood stains were discovered in three locations. First, "there came out of his Nostrils two small Streams of Blood, to the quantity of four Drops." Except for the latter, Hunne's face, chin, doublet, collar, and shirt were free of blood. A large pool was found in a corner at some distance from the body. Finally, much blood was found "within the Flap [pocket?] of the Left side of his Jacket, the latter being folded down over the stain."[7]

Eventually the summoner, Charles Joseph, confessed. According to the statement of his maidservant, a girl named Julian Little, Joseph first swore her to secrecy, then confided, "*I have made away with* Richard Hunne." "*Alas! Master,*" said the Maid, "*He was* reputed an honest Man." Charles answered, "*I have put a Wyre into his Nose.*" Such a weapon could have caused fatal hemorrhage, a lethal brain injury, or both. Joseph added

> *that when* Hunne *was murder'd,* John *the Bell-Ringer carry'd a Wax-Candle up Stairs into the* Lollards *Tower with the Keys of the Door hanging on his Arm: That* Charles [Joseph] *himself went next him, and the Chancellor last: That when they were all got up, they found* Hunne *lying on his bed, upon which the Chancellor said,* Lay Hands on the Thief; *and so they all murder'd him.* Charles *put the Girdle about the Prisoner's Neck; that then John the Bell-Ringer and himself lifted him up, and that the Chancellor pulled the Girdle over the Staple, and so they hang'd him.*

After the wire was thrust firmly into the victim's nose, the body must have rested on the floor long enough for the large pool of blood to have formed. Later, as the dead form was hanged from the staple, a few drops of blood from the nostril fell directly onto the flap on the

7. Hunne had been confined in December in a stone cell, almost certainly unheated. Hence for warmth he wore a jacket over his doublet, which somewhat resembled a modern vest.

left side of the jacket. Finally, as the girdle tightened, the head was displaced to the right. But this is conjecture.

The inquisition states further that

> there was an end of a Wax-Candle, which John the Bell-Ringer saith, he left in the Prison burning with *Hunne* that same *Sunday* at Night that Hunne was murder'd, which Wax-Candle we found sticking upon the stocks[8] fair put out, about seven or eight Foot from the Place where *Hunne* was hang'd; which Candle after our own Opinion was never put out by him, for many likelyhoods which we have perceived. Also at the going up of Master Chancellor into the Lollards Tower, we have good Proof, that there lay on the Stocks a Gown of Murrey [mulberry] or Crimson in grain [color] furred with Shankes [fur from the legs of animals] whose gown it was we could never prove, nor who bore it away.

Note that John the Bell-Ringer said that on Sunday night he left an *end* of wax candle burning on the stocks. When the coroner's jurymen arrived, they noted that the candle had been put out; it could only have burned briefly in Hunne's cell before it was extinguished by his departing visitors or by the prisoner himself. Had the pretended suicidal hanging actually occurred, Hunne would have had to do the deed in the dark or to have waited all night in the blackness of his cell until daylight penetrated—if, indeed, his cell had an opening to the outside world. And how could the prisoner have disposed of the gown trimmed with fur?

Later depositions fill in further details of what happened before and after Hunne's death, details that "put this cruel Murder still past all doubt." The Bishop of London did his best to suppress the whole matter, even appealing for help to Archbishop Wolsey, soon to be made cardinal. It was hoped that Wolsey would ask Henry VIII to intervene. The king compromised by ordering the Attorney General to bring Horsey into court, indicted for murder. He pleaded guilty, was dismissed from office, and retired permanently to Exeter. Hunne's goods, which had been seized, were returned to his children. The fate of Joseph and Spalding is not recorded.

Amid this shameful and sordid affair stand forth the courage, integrity, perception, and good sense of Coroner Barnwell and his twenty-four jurymen. Remember that they were laymen, not medi-

8. The stocks were a wooden framework in which a prisoner was forced to sit, his wrists and ankles confined in front of him, while he was displayed for public ridicule and abuse. It would seem that the apparatus was stored in Hunne's cell.

cal men. Simple citizens of the City of London, they used their eyes and their heads and would not be dissuaded from their verdict, even when the Bishop of London denounced them as "false and perjured caitiffs."

ACCIDENTAL HANGING

A mother who wished to punish her fourteen-year-old daughter tied her to a bedpost about 11:30 A.M. That night the parent found her child in a stooping position, dead. Autopsy showed no marks of violence except a deep indentation, produced by a cord, across the front of the neck. The brain and lungs were congested (*OB,* Dec. 1848: pp. 174–76), a common result of a cervical compression.

SUICIDAL HANGING

A woman's suicidal hanging in 1874 was complicated by the voluntary statement of a young man that he had caused the death—"I have done a murder, I have hung Moggie." He then led a neighbor to the scene. The actual circumstances of death, however, were accurately reconstructed by the police and by surgeons who testified at the trial of the young man for murder.

The rope suspending the victim was attached to a balustrade. Her feet just touched the floor, a fact in itself suggesting suicide. The knot of the running noose was close to her left ear. The noose had produced a bruise, possible only while the victim was still alive, and an oblique indentation on the front and sides, but not back, of the neck. Manual strangulation would have caused a horizontal mark. Her clothing was not disarranged, the furniture was not disturbed, as revealed by the pattern of prints in the dust, and there were no other signs of a struggle. Autopsy disclosed engorgement of brain and lungs with blood and a crushed larynx, all signs of hanging (*OB,* June 1874: pp. 119–25).

This case invites comparison with the Hunne murder. The sixteenth-century affair was, thanks to the coroner and his jury, shown to have been a rather clumsy attempt to make homicide look like suicide. Expert witnesses were able to prove that the 1874 death was suicidal and not, as alleged by a mentally disturbed lover, homicidal.

Both mysteries were solved by hard work, careful observation, and the good sense of lay and expert witnesses.

STRANGULATION BY LIGATURE

The stigmata of strangulation by cord or rope differ in several respects from those of hanging. A sixty-one-year-old woman was found in a bedroom "lying on a box on her back. . . . there was a cord round her neck about the thickness of my little finger—this now produced is it—(looking at it)—it was tied twice round her neck with a knot at the side." Later that day a surgeon examined the body:

> her face was pale, swollen, and livid, her eyes wide open, and staring, blood issuing from her ears and nose, and frothy matter, mixed with blood, coming from the mouth. . . . I noticed two deep circular lines passing round from the front [of the neck] towards the back, marked with discolouration, and only one line at the back of the neck—she died from strangulation, in my judgment. . . . it appeared very improbable from the marks on the neck that she could have effected her destruction herself. . . . the rope must have been tied round the neck during life-time, from the marks and discolouration following from the pulling—I did not perceive any mark, as if made by a knot—if the knot was pulled back, it would be loose from the neck. . . . I examined her hands—there was nothing amounting to the marks I expected to see, as the consequence of the force used to make marks on the neck.

That is, if the victim had *herself* drawn the cord tightly enough to leave marks on the neck, marks would have been expected also on the hands. Note also the important deduction that drawing the knot backward to increase tension would prevent the knot from leaving a mark on the neck (*OB,* Dec. 1845: pp. 178–91).

MANUAL STRANGULATION

Manual strangulation left distinctive marks:

> There was one very remarkable Bruise on her Throat. The Mark on the right Side resembled a Man's Hand—or Fingers; that on the left side was not so large, and was like the Print of a Thumb, and this seemed to be the Death of the Woman. I looked at these Marks, and take them to have been made by a Thumb on one side, and Fingers on the other. (*OB,* July 1740: p. 167)

In 1828 William Burke and William Hare were the defendants in one of Scotland's most notorious murder trials. The woman with whose death they were charged had been strangled so that her body could be sold to an anatomist for dissection. It developed that she was the sixteenth person to have been murdered by the two men for the same commercial purpose. All the victims except the last had been smothered, usually with a pillow, a method calculated to conceal the cause of death. The final corpse had been transported to the dissecting room doubled up, knees to breast and face to knees, in a tea chest.

A post-mortem examination was performed by the Edinburgh surgeons Robert Christison and William Newbigging. The autopsy report (Christison, 1829b) spoke of conjunctival hemorrhages, characteristic of strangulation, and of bruises that had almost certainly been inflicted during life. There was no protrusion of the tongue. The cartilages of the larynx and windpipe had been stretched apart but not fractured; the airway contained mucus. Also observed were hemorrhage under the neck muscles and tearing of the cervical ligaments, although without damage to the cervical vertebrae or spinal cord. At this point the surgeons were uncertain as to whether death was due to the spinal injuries or to manual strangulation.

During the subsequent trial of Burke and Helen McDougal, an accomplice, Hare, by prearrangement, fully implicated Burke. The latter was found guilty, while the jury decided that the charge against Helen McDougal was not proved. Hare went free, and Burke was hanged. Testimony by Hare at the trial, and also a confession written by Burke after his conviction, revealed many additional details and confirmed the cautious conclusions from the autopsy (Douglas, 1973; pp. 74–94, 166–83). Death was indeed by manual strangulation while the intoxicated victim was lying on a bed. It seems almost certain that, as Christison and Newbigging suspected, the cervical trauma occurred later when the corpse was doubled up and forced into the tea chest.

The smothering of infants, as in overlaying, will be considered in the chapter on infanticide.

DROWNING AFTER INJURY

When a body was recovered from a river, pond, or other body of water, it was easy to assume that death was due to drowning. If the corpse showed serious injury, it might be further assumed that drowning occurred during unconsciousness resulting from the injury. But such was not always the case. A surgeon examining the body of a young woman found dead in a canal discovered a severe bruise, such as might have been inflicted with a fist, on the nose; "the blow rendering her insensible, she had not the power to struggle in the water—I should not say that drowning was the immediate cause of death, for I found plenty of air in the lungs, and no water—the body had not imbibed any water" (*OB,* Aug. 1848: pp. 617–21).

The surgeon's observation that drowning had *not* occurred, since the lungs contained air but not water, reflected a reversal of an earlier belief. Until Antoine Lavoisier's discovery in 1776 of the essential role of oxygen in combustion, an observation leading to the first understanding of oxygen's role in respiration, it was generally thought that drowning was fatal because of the *swallowing* of large amounts of water.[9] Gradually the error was corrected. George E. Male, the English pioneer in forensic medicine, seems to have understood the problem:

> The presence of frothy mucus in the mouth and nostrils has, from the days of Ambrose [sic] Paré to the present time, been considered a proof of the body having submersed whilst alive, and is always observed in drowned persons. Water in the stomach is not a proof that the deceased was drowned; it is seldom found there. . . . Larrey[10] found water in the bronchiae [sic] of drowned persons and concludes that it is the cause of death in these cases. When the body is submersed after death, water is never found in the lungs or stomach. (1819: p. 237)

A few years after Male's book appeared P. J. Martin determined that when experimental animals were submerged in muddy water, an earthen residue was found in the bronchi and pulmonary spaces only if the animal was alive when submerged (1826). Nevertheless, twenty-eight years later Dean persisted in the idea that in drowning "the stomach contains a portion, sometimes considerable, of the fluid in which the body is immersed" (1854: p. 433).

9. F. Thomas, 1974. See also the murder of Sarah Stout, chapter 1.
10. Dominique Jean Larrey (1776–1842) was Napoleon's surgeon.

V

Sexual Offenses, Induced Abortion, and Pregnancy

SEXUAL OFFENSES AGAINST FEMALES WERE VARIOUSLY DESCRIBED IN THE Old Bailey indictments as "assaulting," "ravishing," "carnally knowing," "rape" (the term was first used in that court in 1749), and "feloniously and wickedly knowing and abusing." Sexual offenses against males were referred to as "sodomy," "buggery," "attempted sodomy," and "unmentionable offense." There were also a few indictments for "bestiality." Indictments for "indecently assaulting" sometimes did not give the name or sex of the victim; in table 2 these cases are arbitrarily included with rapes.

There was significant medical testimony in 62 of the 144 trials for sexual offenses between 1729 and 1798 (table 2). Medical men were sometimes reluctant or unwilling to appear at all in such cases. When they did enter the witness box, they disagreed or were vague as to the physical signs of defloration, a basic legal question if, as was usual, rape had been alleged.[1] Such hesitation was understandable. Clear evidence of rape resulted in a verdict of guilty; the sentence for this offense was death. Not until the reforms of the early nineteenth century was the penalty reduced to transportation for life.[2]

We know very little about the medical evidence offered in nineteenth-century trials for sexual offenses. Beginning about 1800 medi-

1. The great Morgagni, a leader in eighteenth-century Continental forensic medicine, also found the signs of virginity to be uncertain (1763: pp. 361–78).

2. By 4 and 5 Vict., c. 56, s. 3 (Taylor, 1856: p. 499). Subsequently punishment became much less severe.

Table 2. Old Bailey Trials for Sexual Offenses, 1729–1878

	Offense			
	Against female	Against male	Bestiality	Total
1729–38	18	7		25
1739–48[a]	17	3		20
1749–58	22	4		26
1759–68	14	4		18
1769–78	33	1		34
1779–88	10	1		11
1789–98	10			10
1799–08	3	2		5
1809–18	5	2		7
1819–28	6	1		7
1829–38	72	13		85
1839–48	109	15	4	128
1849–58	65	17	5	87
1859–68	107	23	6	136
1869–78	111	25	11	147
Total	602	118	26	746

[a]Incomplete: some *Sessions Papers* missing.

cal testimony in sex cases was almost always deleted editorially from the *Session Papers,* presumably to avoid offense to readers. A typical record of a trial for a sexual offense in 1811 was as follows:

> JAMES HUGHES was indicted for that he, on the 17th of September, upon Susan Pratchett, Spinster, did make an assault, and her, the said Susan Pratchett, feloniously did ravish and carnally know.
>
> The prisoner called six witnesses, who gave him a good character.
>
> GUILTY—DEATH, aged 26
>
> The prisoner was recommended to his Majesty's mercy, on account of his former good character.[3]
>
> First Middlesex jury, before Mr. Justice Le Blanc. (*OB,* Oct. 1811: p. 437)

The above constitutes the complete account of this trial.

In 1837 Queen Victoria came to the throne, and it may not be a coincidence that by early 1838 rape cases were noted simply with the

3. This meant that he probably would be offered a sentence of transportation to Australia as an alternative to execution.

comment that "the evidence was of a nature unfit for publication."[4] Or an entry in the *Session Papers* would state only that

> 2930. JOHN LEARY was indicted for assaulting Mary Bryan, with intent, &c.
>
> GUILTY. Aged 21.—Confined Twelve Months. (*OB*, Oct. 1839: p. 1058)

> 589. HENRY GODBOLD (27), Feloniously carnally knowing and abusing Louisa Bowyer, aged seven years and four months.
>
> MR. DOUGLAS *conducted the Prosecution.*
>
> GUILTY of the attempt—Two Years' Imprisonment. (*OB*, Oct. 1875: p. 633)

Table 2 shows a conspicuous increase in trials for sexual offenses beginning in the decade 1829–38. It is tempting to speculate as to why this occurred, but hard evidence is lacking. Possible factors include a change in the willingness of victims to report attacks, improved police methods resulting in more frequent arrests, increased effort on the part of prosecutors, and increased frequency of sex crimes as penalties were reduced.

An eighteenth-century obstacle to the prosecution of some persons accused of sexual offenses was the unwillingness of many judges to administer the oath to young children. If they could not be sworn, these victims might not be allowed to testify: "*The child being so young, and not knowing the nature of an oath, could not be examined. . . . There being no other evidence against the prisoner than hearsay from the child's mouth, it was not judged sufficient; he was therefore acquitted* (*OB*, May 1754: p. 216).

Seventy-three trials for sexual offenses were recorded in which expert testimony was offered. Of the victims, seventy-one were females (their ages are recorded in table 3). More than half were under the age of eleven years; it is not clear why cases of alleged rape of adults seldom came to trial.

Diagnosis of defloration was made by a midwife, apothecary, or medical man. Sometimes the examiner concluded that rape had not occurred. A fourteen-year-old alleged victim, suspected of prostitution, got little sympathy:

> I am an apothecary and surgeon; I examined the prosecutrix.
>
> What did you observe?—I observed that she had a very great discharge, of a bad colour, yellow.

4. Evidence in at least three infanticide cases (see next chapter) was suppressed for the same reason (*OB*, Sept. 1850: p. 629; May 1851: p. 63; Dec. 1876: p. 221).

Table 3. Ages of Female Victims in Old Bailey Trials for Sexual Offenses

Age	No.	Age	No.
2 yr.	2	13 yr.	3
3	2	14	4
4	4	15	2
5	1	16	2
6	3	17	1
7	1	18	2
8	9	Adult	6
9	10	Not	
10	10	known	1
11	5	Total	71
12	3		

What do you mean, the foul disorder?—Yes.

Was there a great laceration of the parts?—No, I did not observe anything of that . . .

Did you examine the man?—He seemed to have no disorder at all, there appeared nothing.

Court to Jury. Gentlemen, then there is an end of this business, indeed there was an end of it before.

NOT GUILTY. (*OB*, July 1783: p. 726)

Not only were some accused persons under the influence of alcohol at the times of their alleged offenses, but the victim might also be intoxicated; the drinking of spirits by persons of all ages, young children included, particularly in the first half of the eighteenth century, was on an almost unbelievable scale. A man was indicted "for Ravishing and Carnally Knowing" an eleven-year-old girl on 11 April 1735. A midwife examined her on 17 April and found signs of sexual abuse. The girl had gone to the shop of the accused "with two or three of my Play-fellows to drink a Dram." Said another witness, a woman, "this girl and another came in for a Quartern[5] of Gin. . . . She came two or three times that Day for Gin." A third woman told the court: "I saw the girl on the fifteenth of *April*. She said the Prisoner had had to do with her, to be sure. I asked her why she did not cry out. *Because,* says she, *he gave me a Dram of Anniseed, and I shall have a pretty baby of my own*

5. A quarter of a pint.

to nurse, and that will be better than crying out (*OB*, Oct. 1735: pp. 161–62).

Venereal diseases were incompletely understood in the eighteenth and nineteenth centuries. The symptoms of syphilis and gonorrhea were confused,[6] a situation that was not helped by the eminent John Hunter's conclusion, based on an experiment and accepted for long afterward, that the two diseases were one and the same (Herman, 1978). Transmission of a venereal disease was recognized as a possible result of a sexual assault. It often happened that the molestation of a child was first disclosed when an adult, usually a parent, noticed the appearance of painful symptoms or the soiling of underclothes. The discovery might not take place until days or even weeks after the attack, the child having remained silent through ignorance and fright.

There seems little doubt that some young girls were assaulted because of a widespread myth (Hovorka and Kronfeld, 1909: *2*, 151) that venereal disease would be cured by coitus with a virgin. The case of an eleven-year-old is an example. A surgeon who examined the girl two days after she was attacked found symptoms of venereal infection in both the victim and the accused.

> *Q.* I will ask you a question for the sake of the public, and enlightening the public mind upon this subject; is it possible for a man, having a venereal taint of this sort, to receive any benefit from connexion with a child?—*A.* It is an extremely false idea.
>
> *Court.* This idea cannot be too well understood, because many poor miserable wretches have that notion?—*A.* I should suppose quite the reverse. . . .
>
> *Court.* That has been the uniform answer of every surgeon that I ever heard. (*OB,* Feb. 1796: pp. 304–07)

There is no indication that transmission of a venereal disease was per se a crime.

Early-nineteenth-century writers on forensic medicine discussed sexual offenses chiefly in terms of the physical signs of defloration and rape (Farr, 1819: pp. 24–27; Beck and Beck, 1835: pp. 113–15). Burrows commented: "Physicians and legislators are much divided in their consideration of the crime of rape. Some deny the possibility of the perpetration of such a crime. The proofs of its commission are few and uncertain; and perhaps there is no accusation in support of which our courts of law have shewn more caution and jealousy in admitting testimony than in such charges" (1831: p. 17).

6. See, for example, Beckett, 1718; Waugh, 1973.

However, the remarkable Alfred Swaine Taylor devoted eighteen pages in the 1856 edition of his *Medical Jurisprudence* to a discussion of rape and other sex offenses. He discussed the physical signs to be observed in the victim, then went on to review the Continental literature on the identification of seminal stains, citing Chevallier's important paper of 1834. Taylor pointed out that sperm from a stain may be identified under the microscope, describing his own observations as well as those of others (1856: pp. 499–516; Smyth, 1980: pp. 193–94).

INDUCED ABORTION

One can only speculate about the incidence of induced abortion in England before the nineteenth century. The act seems not to have been obvious or frequent enough to have aroused comment. Deliberate abortion was for a long time not a serious offense in the eyes of the law. Said the eminent jurist Sir Matthew Hale (1609–76), "an infant in its mother's womb, not being *in rerum natura,* is not considered as a person who can be killed within the description of murder; and therefore if a woman, being quick or great with child, takes any potion, or if a person shakes her, whereby the child within her is killed, it is not murder or manslaughter" (quoted by W. Hutchinson, 1820). In 1765 Blackstone commented: "For if a woman is quick with child, and by a potion or otherwise killeth it in her womb; or if anyone beat her, whereby the child dieth in her body, and she is delivered of a dead child; this, though not murder, was by the ancient law homicide or manslaughter. But the modern law doth not look upon this offense in quite so atrocious a light but merely as a heinous misdemeanor" (1872: Book I, p. 129).

In 1803 the Ellenborough Act[7] first made induced abortion a statutory offense (L. A. Parry, 1932: p. 86); it provided that

> if any Person or Persons . . . shall wilfully and maliciously administer to, or cause to be administered to, or taken by any Woman, any Medicine, Drug, or other Substance or Thing whatsoever, or shall use or employ, or cause to be used or employed, any Instrument or other Means whatsoever, with Intent thereby to cause or procure the Miscarriage of any Woman not being, or not being proved to be, quick with Child[8] at the Time of administering such Things or using such

7. 45 Geo. 3, c. 58. For a review of abortion in nineteenth century Britain see Sauer, 1978.

8. The fetus was said to be "quick" when its movements could be felt.

> Means . . . shall be and are declared guilty of felony, and shall be liable to be fined, imprisoned, set in and upon the Pillory, publicly or privately whipped . . . or transported beyond the sea for any term not exceeding fourteen years. (Raithby, 1823: p. 65)

The act went on to decree that administration of medicines or drugs *after* quickening to procure an abortion was punishable by death.

The Offences against the Person Act, passed in 1828, made it illegal to procure abortion with a drug or medicine or by any means (9 Geo. 4, c. 31; Statutes, 1828: p. 104). In 1837 the law on abortion was changed, and capital punishment was abolished as a penalty for this offense (1 Vict., c. 85). The new statute stated that

> whosoever, with Intent to procure the Miscarriage of any Woman, shall unlawfully administer to her or cause to be taken by her any Poison or other noxious Thing, or shall unlawfully use any Instrument or other Means whatsoever, with the like Intent, shall be guilty of Felony, and being convicted thereof, shall be liable, at the Discretion of the Court, to be transported beyond the Seas for the Term of his or her natural Life, or for any Term, not less than Fifteen Years, or to be imprisoned for any Term not exceeding Three Years. (Statutes, 1837: p. 360)

Dr. A. T. Thomson, lecturing on medical jurisprudence at the University of London in 1836, gave it as his opinion that "mechanical means . . . are as frequently employed as medicine to cause criminal abortion" (1837: p. 629). The scattered evidence available suggests that professional abortionists were few, that charges were rarely brought, or convictions obtained, for "feticide," and that the crime itself may have been infrequently committed up to at least the latter part of the nineteenth century.[9]

By that time attitudes were changing. Woodman and Tidy in 1877 solemnly warned, although without citing any evidence whatsoever, that "it is to be feared that criminal abortion is on the increase in England. It is fearfully prevalent in the United States, and was so formerly in France. The "Free-lovers," and other so-called religious sects of America, and some of the sexless things known as advocates of Women's Rights in England, have at different times openly and unblushingly advocated the practice" (1877: p. 633).

One trial for the instrumental procurement of an abortion was encountered in the *Sessions Papers*. In 1848 a thirty-two-year-old unmarried woman went to a Mrs. Dryden, who "said it would be all

9. Hutchinson, 1820: p. 97; Thomson, 1837: p. 625; Sauer, 1978: pp. 83–84.

right, if I would pay her 4*s*., and which I gave her; she gave me a box of pills and a bottle of stuff, which did not have the expected effect." Mrs. Dryden then took her to a Mrs. Lindfield, who "told me to lay on the bed on my left side; she then performed an operation by some instrument, which had some holes at the end." Neither this nor a second attempt with the instrument were successful. The young woman became ill, and died ten days later.

The abortionists were arrested and charged with murder. The police searched Mrs. Dryden's house and "found herbs there, and a small portion of Savin. . . . at Dryden's I found these two bills, and two cards. (*These were headed, Mrs. Lindfield, Midwife, Dentist, and Practical Herbalist, &c., and contained a long list of herbs, ointments, &c., for the cure of various disorders; and the words 'retirement for ailing females.'*" At Mrs. Lindfield's house the police discovered a document certifying that she "has diligently attended a course of my lectures on midwifery, and the diseases of women and children; and practised the same under my inspection.—24th May, 1821—Henry Gore Clough, M.D., Accoucheur and Physician (to several institutions), Professor and Lecturer on the Science of Midwifery, Berners-street."

A surgeon who had attended the victim in her last illness testified to "great constitutional disturbance," lower abdominal pain, and signs of a miscarriage:

> (*The particulars of the post-mortem examination—and of the cross-examination of this witness, were not of a nature fit for publication; he attributed the death to inflammation of the uterus, arising from abortion, but stated that the injury which appeared to have produced the inflammation was not occasioned by the use of the catheter.*)

The prisoners were found not guilty (*OB*, Oct. 1848: pp. 1079–84).

The administration of drugs to procure abortions is discussed in the chapter on poison.

PREGNANCY

Pregnancy was an important complication of several homicides. In April 1786 a woman in her sixth month of gestation had a drunken quarrel one Saturday night and was severely bruised. She became ill and three days later delivered a fetus, which soon succumbed. The next day, very sick, she was examined by a surgeon, who determined that she was dying of typhus fever.

Post-mortem examination did not include opening the body. The miscarriage was ascribed to injuries received during the fight, the woman's death to typhus fever and the inflammation and mortification which allegedly followed. The court sought enlightenment from the medical witnesses:

> This species of fevers, is that the species of fever that ordinarily attends child-bearing?—Generally, it first arises from an inflammatory fever, which is what we call a puerperal fever.
>
> Where the party is delivered on Tuesday, and is in a dying state on Thursday, is that the puerperal fever?—I look upon it, that this fever was brought on by passion. . . .
>
> An inflammatory fever that degenerates into a putrid fever, I should apprehend would require some time?—Not much, my Lord.
>
> These puerperal fevers are brought on I suppose by a variety of causes?—Yes: either from pains of delivery or the state of discharges after delivery.

From this display of etiological confusion it is difficult to determine much more than that a fatal septicemia seems to have coincided with or followed the premature and perhaps traumatic delivery.

By now the judge had had enough. He began his summing up with a castigation of the witnesses:

> *Court to Jury.* Gentlemen, the prisoner stands indicted for the wilful murder of Ann Rose. . . . the circumstances of the case, as well as we can collect them from witnesses, who either do not speak so correctly as one would wish them to do, or have their reasons for not stating accurately the whole that is past, are these. (*Here the learned Judge summed up the evidence and then added.*) . . . Upon these circumstances you are to say, in the first place, whether this woman's death is at all imputable to any thing that was done by the prisoner, on the Saturday night. . . . the deceased appears from all I can collect to the contrary to have been in health, before this affray happened;. . .upon the whole of the evidence, though undoubtedly these fevers are no uncommon consequences of all kinds of birth natural as well as premature, yet, when you find the woman does not appear to be in ill health before a premature birth, brought on soon after this affray, I think you can hardly doubt much, but that the affray which happened on Saturday night, did contribute to bring on that premature birth, which was followed by this fever, of which the woman died. . . . But the points for your consideration are, whether this woman's death has been brought on by this affray, that happened on Saturday evening; and if it was, whether, in the course of this affray any blame is imputable to the prisoner.

The jury found her guilty of manslaughter (*OB,* April 1786: pp. 627–36).

Once again, one observes a familiar medicolegal problem—when a physical assault, nonlethal in itself, initiates a series of results, the last of which is fatal, to what extent is the assailant guilty? Obviously the jury's decision largely depended on its understanding of the expert medical testimony. In the present case, the previously healthy Mrs. Rose apparently was not fatally injured by her fall. Did the latter cause the premature delivery? Allegedly so. Did the fatal illness, variously described as putrid fever, inflammatory fever, mortification, and puerperal fever, in turn result from the premature birth or, as suggested, from anger, "from pains of delivery or the state of discharges after delivery"? At this point in their deliberations, if not before, the unfortunate jurymen must have realized that they, though laymen, had been handed a medical problem which the surgeons were unable to resolve. Unlike the expert witnesses, the jurymen could not equivocate.

We can ponder two further possibilities in the Lewis case. One is that an autopsy might have shown that the victim received a fatal internal injury *when* she fell. The other is that the deadly septicemia might have been present, as yet undetected, *before* Mrs. Rose was injured.

There was one more act to the drama. No sooner had sentence been pronounced on Frances Lewis for the manslaughter of Ann Rose than the prisoner was tried again for manslaughter, this time in the death of Mrs. Rose's prematurely delivered baby. But the judge dealt speedily with this charge:

> *Court to jury.* Gentlemen, this is, you easily perceive, another method of bringing the case before you; I shall recommend to you in this case, to find a general verdict of not guilty; it is a great deal too much to charge, on the circumstances of the child being alive, the death of the child to the prisoner at the bar, in any shape at all; to be sure the child perished merely in consequence of a premature birth; therefore publick justice is satisfied with what you have done already, and it would be an improper verdict to find her guilty.

The jury acceded to the direction of the court (*OB,* April 1786: p. 636).

VI

Infanticide

IN 1624 A HARSH LAW WAS ENACTED BY JAMES I TO COMBAT THE DEADLY sin of infanticide (21 Jac. 1, c. 27):

> Whereas many lewd women that have been delivered of bastard children, to avoid their shame, and to escape punishment, do secretly bury or conceal the death of their children, and after, if the child be found dead, the said women do alledge, that the said child was born dead; whereas it falleth out sometimes (although hardly it is to be proved) that the said child or children were murthered by the said women, their lewd mothers, or by their assent or procurement:
>
> For the preventing therefore of this great mischief, be it enacted by the authority of this present parliament, That if any woman after one month next ensuring the end of the session of parliament be delivered of any issue of her body, male or female, which being born alive, should by the laws of this realm be a bastard, and that she endeavour privately, either by drowning or secret burying thereof, or any other way, either by her self or the procuring of others, so to conceal the death thereof, as that it may not come to light, whether it were born alive or not, but be concealed: in every such case the said mother so offending shall suffer death as in case of murther, except such mother can make proof by one witness at the least, that the child (whose death was by her so intended to be concealed) was born dead. (Pickering, 1763: 7, 298)

The statute was exceptional in English law in that, in effect, guilt of the accused was presumed until innocence was proven. As Blackstone later remarked, the act "savours pretty strongly of severity in making the concealment of the death almost conclusive evidence of the child's being murdered by the mother." But, he adds, "it has of late years been usual with us in England, upon trials for this offence, to require some sort of presumptive evidence that the child was born alive, before the other constrained presumption (that the child whose death is concealed was therefore killed by its parent) is admitted to convict the prisoner" (1872: *4*, 198). Malcolmson points out that the emphasis of the law is on concealment of birth, less difficult to prove than infanticide (1977: pp. 196–97).

A case tried in 1688 at the Old Bailey, while it does not involve much forensic medical testimony, serves well to illustrate the operation of the act of 1624:

> *Sinah Jones* of the Parish of St. *Mary Woolnoth,* was Indicted for Murdering her Bastard Male Child, on the Eighteenth of *December* last, being Saturday Night, by stopping its Breath with a Cloath put in its Mouth; she being a Servant in the House of Mr. *Cousins.* The Evidence against her was plain, the Nurse, the Chair-woman, the Midwife, the Master and his Servant, all deposing, that she denying the Key, they broke open her Trunk, where they all saw the Child Dead, wrapped up in a Cloath, with a Rag in the Mouth of it, as big as a Handkerchief, and that the Child being something Warm, they tried all they could to recover Life in it, but to no purpose. The Prisoner said little for herself, but that she knew nothing of the Cloath in the Mouth of the Child, and that she had not her Senses, and was Light-headed. Then the Statute was read to her, wherein, If the Child be found Dead and Concealed, though it were so Born, the Person Concealing it, shall suffer Death as in case of Murder, except she can prove by one Witness at least that the Child so Concealed was born Dead. Upon full Evidence, she was brought in guilty of Murder. (*OB,* Jan. 1688: p. 1)

Blackstone was not alone in his view that the act of 1624 was inhumane. William Hunter in 1783 published an eloquent defense of the hapless mothers, often lonely servant girls, and commented vigorously "On the Uncertainty of the Signs of Murder, in the Case of Bastard Children" (1783). Others also attacked the law (Malcolmson, p. 197), and it was abolished by the Ellenborough Act of 1803.[1] This statute additionally provided that mothers of illegitimate offspring if acquitted of murder could instead be convicted of concealment of birth. The maximum penalty for concealment was set at two years in prison. Now a compassionate jury could by its verdict avoid the death penalty but still not let an act of infanticide go without punishment, a merciful alternative which at once found favor (table 4).

An interesting point has been made about the Ellenborough Act.

1. 43 Geo. 3, c. 58; Raithby, 1823: pp. 63–66.

Table 4. Old Bailey Infanticide Trials with Expert Medical Testimony, 1729–1878

	Charge		Verdict				Sentence	
	Murder	Manslaughter	Not guilty	Murder	Manslaughter	Concealment	Death	Prison
1729–38	9		4	5			5	
1739–48	4	1	4	1			1	
1749–58	5		4	1			1	
1759–68	7		6	1			1	
1769–78	4		4					
1779–88	5		5					
1789–98	1		1					
1799–08	7		4			3		3
1809–18	13		9	1		3	1	3
1819–28	6	1	6	1			1	
1829–38	7	3	3		2	5		7
1839–48	15		5		1	9		10
1849–58	10	5	11		2	2		4
1859–68	16	1	3	2	2	10	2	12
1869–78	5	2	2	1	2	2	1	4
Total	114	13	71	13	9	34	13	43

Note: Not included are two cases counted as assaults (table 2), two cases with no verdict, and one case that was respited.

"The provisional presumption of our Common Law, and by Statute since Lord Ellenborough's Act . . . is that a child is born dead. . . . The fact of Live-birth must be established by valid evidence, usually *res ipsa loquitur*"[2] (Atkinson, 1904: p. 134). Thus to prove infanticide it was necessary first to establish that the child had lived. As we shall see, this could be very difficult.

By the Offences against the Person Act of 1828, the law was extended to make concealment of birth by any mother, married or not, an offense (9 Geo. 4, c. 31; Statutes, 1828: p. 104). The Offences against the Person Act of 1861 decreed that concealment of the dead baby by *any* person, not simply the mother, was a felony (24 & 25 Vict., c. 100). The law also continued to make available as an alternative to a verdict of murder the finding of concealment of the body (Rickards, 1861: p. 439).

Jurists, the press, and at least a segment of the medical profession in the 1860s and 1870s were disturbed by the fact that infanticide trials almost never resulted in a conviction for murder (Ryan, 1862: pp. 48–62; Langer, 1974). Davies quotes figures for Britain indicating that the "total number of committals for trial for concealment" rose from 44 in 1834 to 522 in 1857–61. No woman had been hanged for infanticide since 1849.[3] Sauer (1978) and Behlmer (1979) summarize data from official reports that confirm this trend. Malcolmson notes sixty-one trials for infanticide at the Old Bailey between 1730 and 1774; forty-six of the women charged were found not guilty.[4] Statistics on infanticide in past centuries are usually unsatisfactory both because of certain inadequacies of the surviving records and because many homicides of the newborn undoubtedly were not discovered. Thomas Wakley, for example, the vigorous and enlightened Coroner of West Middlesex, estimated in about 1862 that in London two hundred infanticides went undetected annually (Ryan, 1862: p. 79).

Those guilty of infanticide, their victims, and the act itself had certain distinguishing characteristics. Newborn babies were nearly always killed by women, usually their mothers, and death commonly occurred within a few minutes to an hour or so after delivery. Death might be due to trauma or to neglect. The numbers of boy and girl babies killed were roughly equal. The majority of mothers were

2. "The thing speaks for itself."

3. Davies, 1937: p. 218. For further discussions of the law on abortion and infanticide see the excellent reviews of Atkinson, 1904; Davies, 1937; and Hull and Hoffer, 1981.

4. Note that table 4 includes only infanticide trials with medical testimony.

young, poor servants, shop girls, dressmakers, and the like. There was little or no evidence, before and during the trial, of interest and support from the accused's family; she was likely one of the great numbers of males and females who left home and came into London seeking work (Malcolmson, 1977: p. 192; K. Clarke, 1980).

Illegitimate pregnancy placed a woman in a desperate position.[5] Concealment of her plight became increasingly difficult in a household or shop amid other women. If her pregnancy were discovered, she faced shame, loss of employment, and little or no prospect of a character reference to support a search for new work. If she "lived in," she was cast into the street unless her mistress was kinder than most. Society might condone the unchaste man but not the unchaste woman.[6] If the pregnant girl did find a job, it would be menial and she could be easily exploited. Too often there remained for her only a life on the fringe of the law or beyond it. A woman who resorted to infanticide had the further immediate problem of concealment of the body and of disposal of bloody linen and telltale stains, together with continuing anxiety that any trace might betray her.

An illustrative case occurred in 1784. Elizabeth Curtis was charged with murdering her newborn child. At her trial counsel, summarizing testimony given at the inquest, stated that

> she was a servant to Mrs. Soy, who kept the Blue-Posts. . . . her mistress observed that she was with child, and she told her she suspected her situation; the young woman denied the charge. . . . a Mrs. Baker a midwife was sent for, and when she came she observed to the young woman, that she either was or lately had been brought to bed, and desired her to confess; the young woman then said, it is true, the child is wrapped up in a napkin there on the side of the bed; she said, she was ashamed to own it; she was then asked whether the child was born alive or not; she said, the child was still born, and had never been born alive; she was then asked, whether she had provided any things in case the child had been born alive to put it in; she said, she had, and they very properly examined the drawers, and found amongst the young woman's clothes, some things proper for the child.

5. For a discussion of the social background see Langer, 1974; Wrightson, 1975; Malcolmson, 1977; Damme, 1978; Sauer, 1978; Behlmer, 1979; Greenwald and Greenwald, 1981.

6. Even if the father could be located and successfully prosecuted, under the law he was at most liable for small payments for support of the mother and her baby during the first nineteen weeks after delivery. And the mother paid all the legal costs (F. B. Smith, 1979: p. 70).

Such a search for baby clothes was common. If found, they were often regarded as evidence that the mother had desired the baby to live. But a woman planning infanticide might lay away baby clothes as a ruse.

Then a surgeon and "man midwife" testified that he had asked the mother "if the child was born alive; I asked her if the child cried, she said not; I asked her if she felt the child move, she said no; I asked her if she did not use a knife to cut the navel string; she said she did not, she said she tore it. I should not suppose it was born alive; my opinion is, that the child died in the birth for want of assistance" (*OB,* Sept. 1784: pp. 1221–23).

Hemorrhage from the umbilical cord could occur if the cut or broken cord were not ligated. If a dead newborn with signs of massive bleeding from the cord were discovered and if the birth had been unattended, the mother might be held responsible for causing the death by neglect or malice. Male pointed out that fatal umbilical hemorrhage did not always follow failure to ligate the severed cord and that the cords of newborn animals were not ligated. He also warned, "An artful woman may let the child die of haemorrhage, and then apply the ligature; this may be ascertained by the emptiness of the veins and heart, and the small quantity of blood found on dissection" (1819: p. 187). Paris and Fonblanque (1823: *3,* pp. 126–27) and Ryan (1831: p. 161) concurred.

Fatal incised wounds in infants as described at the Old Bailey were all in the neck region. If little blood was found, it was usually assumed that the assault had occurred elsewhere (*OB,* Dec. 1778: pp. 56–60). After observing a razor wound, the surgeon estimated that the injury "had been inflicted before death—the flesh would present a different appearance if the wound was inflicted after death" (*OB,* July 1863: p. 345), a significant point. Scissors made an irregular opening—an "incised wound cut by scissars and notched." Counsel suggested that the injury might have occurred when the mother used scissors to attempt to release an umbilical cord wound tightly around the baby's neck, a contingency that could indeed arise, but the surgeon pointed out that the wound could scarcely have been accidental, being more than an inch deep (*OB,* April 1808: pp. 210–13).

In 1800 a servant girl was discovered to have delivered herself. The infant, still alive but bleeding from the nose and mouth, was found under a pile of soiled clothing. It succumbed in an hour or two. The autopsy revealed a wound, seemingly done with a rather dull object, far back on the tongue. Counsel suggested that the mother might accidentally have injured the baby during delivery:

> *M. Knapp*. *Q*. When the head is born, would it not have been natural for the mother, delivering herself in that rude manner, to grasp the throat?—*A*. Certainly.
>
> *Q*. But suppose, instead of grasping the throat, she had, with a strong nail, put her finger in the mouth?—*A*. Then she would have wounded the palate, and not the tongue. . . .
>
> *Court*. *Q*. What kind of laceration of the tongue was this?—*A*. It was about an inch and a half in length, across the tongue, and a quarter of an inch in depth. (*OB*, Jan. 1800: pp. 77–82)

A finger inserted deep into the baby's mouth, due to the curve and narrow diameter of the mouth and throat, could only enter with its *palmar* side toward the tongue; the fingernail would lie away from the tongue. Thus the wound must almost certainly have been made by the end of an instrument such as a knife or scissors blade, and therefore the wounding was deliberate and not accidental. Nevertheless, the prisoner was found not guilty.

LUNG FLOTATION

A classical test to determine whether a dead infant had ever breathed was to remove its lungs and place them in water.[7] Dense, uninflated fetal lung tissue was expected to sink, inflated lungs to float. A surgeon, called in to examine the recently delivered body of a dead baby, explained:

> There were no marks of violence about the child. . . . On the Tuesday, by order of the Coroner, I proceeded to make an internal examination—I first opened the chest, and took out the lungs and the heart attached—I found that they floated—the lungs were sufficiently buoyant to sustain the weight of the heart. . . . I then cut the lungs into a number of small pieces, and carefully compressed them, still every piece floated. . . . I believe the lungs of an infant could not be inflated to such an extent during the progress of delivery. (*OB*, Oct. 1847: pp. 1171–75)

The lung flotation test, which emerged during the seventeenth century, has been erroneously ascribed to Galen (Kühn, 1822: bk. 15, chap. 6, p. 243). But it appears that his contribution was simply to

7. Lung flotation was also known as the hydrostatic test or *Docimasia pulmonum hydrostatica*. Brittain has published a comprehensive historical review (1963). See also Friedreich, 1844; Ackerknecht and Kozelka, 1950: p. 1295; S. Smith, 1954; Forbes, 1978: pp. 46–47.

observe that upon respiration at birth "the fleshy substance of the lung is transformed from something red, heavy, and dense to a material white, light, and loose in texture." In 1626 Spigelius confirmed Galen's observation. Thomas Bartholin, a Danish anatomist, observed that the lung substance "in a Child in the Womb is compact and thick; so that being cast into Water it sinks, which the Lungs of grown person will not do" (1663: bk. 2, chap. 9, p. 117). Four years later Johann Swammerdam of Leyden noted in his doctoral thesis that in a fetus just before birth "the lungs are compacted on themselves and the chest is expanded, without any denser air inside between the lungs and ribs" (1667).

According to one source, Karel Rayger, like Bartholin a seventeenth-century anatomist, first proposed the use of the hydrostatic test in the forensic medical investigation of infanticide. Said Rayger, "I believe it [the test] an indubitable proof for crimes of infanticide. . . whether the infant died in utero or later, after birth, was strangled or killed in some way" (1675; cited by Nemec, 1973: p. 169; 1976: pp. 51–52). About the same time Johann Schreyer, a Silesian physician, applied the test in investigating the case of a fifteen-year-old farm girl accused of killing her baby. The lungs sank and the prisoner was acquitted.[8]

Numerous authors questioned the validity of the test. It was suggested that a feeble newborn living only for a few hours might not inflate its lungs sufficiently for them to be able to float. Artificial respiration or the gases of putrefaction, on the other hand, might expand the lungs of a stillborn.[9]

William Hunter, M.D., elder brother of John Hunter, was Physician Extraordinary to the Queen, Fellow of the Royal Society, Member of the Royal Academy of Sciences of Paris, and a prominent London accoucheur.[10] Stirred by the problems of infanticide and the unwed mother, he produced a remarkable essay, "On the Uncertainty of the Signs of Murder, in the Case of Bastard Children," read posthumously to the Medical Society in July 1784 and published the same year (1784; W. Cummin, 1836: p. 23). The paper was not only the first original contribution in English to the field of forensic medicine but an important, if somewhat emotional, statement of the prob-

8. Nemec, 1973: p. 157; Garrison, 1929: p. 272; Brittain, 1963: p. 190.

9. Continental observers who doubted the reliability of the flotation test included Bohn, 1711: pp. 171–84; von Haller, 1721; and Morgagni, 1769: b. 2, letter 19, article 45.

10. The term *obstetrician* was not coined until 1828.

lems relating to the proof of still and live birth. It must be recalled that at this time the statute of James I regarding infanticide and concealment of birth had not yet been abolished.

Hunter's essay is based, he says, on lectures to his students. After referring to his extensive experience in treating and delivering women and to his resultant "knowing a good deal of female characters," he comes eloquently to the defense of unmarried "women who are pregnant without daring to avow their situation . . . and generally are less criminal than the world imagines. In most of these cases the father of the child is really criminal, often cruelly so; the mother is weak, credulous, and deluded." A woman who delivers her baby alone is terrified and irrational. If under such circumstances she turns to suicide, thereby ending also the life of her unborn baby, her act is not calculated murder but one "committed under a phrenzy from despair."

Should she be arrested and brought to court, grave responsibility rests on the medical men called to testify. Hunter is blunt about the shortcomings of some experts:

> But danger, in the cases of which we are now treating, may arise from the evidence and opinions given by physical people, who are called in to settle questions in science, which judges and jurymen are supposed not to know with accuracy. In general I am afraid too much has been left to our decision. Many of our profession are not so conversant with science as the world may think: and some of us are disposed to grasp at authority in a public examination, by giving a quick and decided opinion, where it should have been guarded with doubt; a character which no man should be ambitious to acquire, who in his profession is presumed every day to be deciding nice questions upon which the life of a patient may depend.
>
> To form a solid judgment about the birth of a new-born child, from the examination of its body, a professional man should have seen many new-born children, both stillborn and such as had outlived their birth a short time only: and he should have dissected, or attended the dissections of a number of bodies in the different stages of advancing putrefaction. I have often seen various common and natural appearances, both internal and external, mistaken for marks of a violent death.

Hunter tells how the physician may fail to understand post-mortem skin changes and settling of the blood, and appearances of swelling, reddening, or blackening which can give a false impression of strangulation.

Then the shrewd Scot turns to the lung flotation test, rehearsing the difficulties mentioned by other writers. Even, he says, if all these objections are borne in mind and the test is conducted with great care, a positive result "cannot amount to more than a ground of suspicion, and therefore we should not determine a question, otherwise doubtful, between an acquitted, or an ignominious death. . . . If in the case of a concealed birth, it be clearly made out that a child had breathed, may we infer that it was murdered? Certainly not. It is certainly a circumstance . . . which amounts only to suspicion." Hunter asserts that he knows from his own experience that if a newborn dies after one gasp, the lungs will float. A child may respire as soon as its head emerges from the birth canal but succumb before delivery is complete, even when skilled assistance is at hand. Or a newborn may die in the first minute or first hour after birth. Even after a normal delivery the baby may not survive if the mother is unconscious and no one else is present to raise the infant and clear the air passages.

In the eighteenth century other tests for live birth were put forward,[11] only to fall into disrepute.[12] Probably the best known was Ploucquet's, which was based on the ratios of body weight to inflated and uninflated lung weights (1786). In later years it was shown that normal newborn organ and body weights vary so widely as to make their comparative ratios useless. Taylor, with characteristic thoroughness, reviewed the literature on the flotation test and conducted his own experiments, concluding that it "is only capable of determining that respiration has taken place; it cannot show whether that process was established during birth, or afterwards." Again, "the hydrostatic test is no more capable of showing that a child has *been born alive or dead,* than it is of proving whether it has been murdered, or has died from natural causes" (1838: pp. 571, 587).

Careful examination of the lung itself gradually supplanted the flotation test. A certain Buttner, according to Fodéré (1813: p. 481), was the first to suggest that when the gases of putrefaction had expanded the lungs of a stillborn, "the arteries as well as the veins of these artificially inflated lungs remain empty and in a state of collapse, as one can convincingly show by dissection." Guy looked for the characteristic "bright vermillion-coloured groups of air-cells scattered over the surface" of the lung as an indication whether respiration

11. Beck, 1817: pp. 50–65; 1842: pp. 1–6; Webster, 1824: pp. 17–20, Dunglison, 1827: pp. 103–08; Burrows, 1831: pp. 17–18; Cummin, 1836: pp. 32–46; Watson, 1842: pp. 290–94: Ogston, 1878: pp. 229–38.

12. Percival, 1794: p. 63; Male, 1819: pp. 189–92; M. Ryan, 1831: pp. 162–63, 171; Williams, 1835: pp. 102–09.

or artificial inflation had occurred (1845: pp. 150–53; Guy and Ferrier, 1875: pp. 90–93), an observation in keeping with modern procedure.[13]

Flotation of the lungs is not now considered to be a useful method when employed as the only criterion for live birth (Polson and Gee, 1973: pp. 538–39; Rentoul and Smith, 1973: pp. 404–05).[14] But, as Brittain has pointed out, this and other tests "are nonetheless important in the history of legal medicine. Each was an attempt to use medicine for the benefit of law, to develop science specifically to the furtherance of justice" (1963).

STRANGULATION, SUFFOCATION, AND DROWNING

A surgeon who examined the body of a dead newborn found signs of strangulation, observing

> a mark round the neck . . . and under this mark I found extravasated blood in the cellular membrane, under the skin. . . . it had every appearance of having been born alive—of having breathed. . . . the mark [on the neck] was much smaller than I consider the navel string would have made; the tongue protruded from the mouth. . . . the vessels of the brain were filled with blood, and there was a spot of extravasated blood on the left side of the brain. (*OB*, May 1832: pp. 511–13)

Here is evidence of a relatively careful post-mortem examination. The surgeon considered, but rejected, the possibility that the child might have been choked by the umbilical cord. Extravasation of blood under the ligature and on the surface of the brain and protrusion of the tongue were significant.

Suffocation occurred in a variety of locations, most commonly in a privy or "vault" where the baby had been dropped. Sometimes the mother asserted that she had unknowingly delivered the infant while

13. See, for example, Simpson, 1975: p. 162.

14. The definition of live birth has long provided a medicolegal dilemma. In 1854 Amos Dean, Professor of Medical Jurisprudence at Albany Medical College, published an interesting textbook, written in catechismal form, which includes a section on the investigation of infanticide. Dean asks, "Was the child born alive? . . . What is the meaning of the term *born alive*?" The answer, he says, is that the infant must have survived until completely delivered, and the necessary changes must have occurred to establish an independent circulation. It is not necessary that the umbilical cord have been divided. Dean, who was also a counselor at law, supplies a court decision to support each of his medical criteria (1854: p. 140).

seated in the privy, a story which, however unlikely, was difficult to disprove.

Suffocation, as William Hunter had suggested (1783), might also occur by accident after delivery if the mother were unconscious and no other adult were present to assist the child. In a case of this kind, the surgeon who performed the autopsy noted that the lungs

> appeared to have been extended and inflated with air, and were of a bright red appearance—that indicates that the lungs must have been in contact with oxygen or atmospheric air, and that blood must have circulated, that the child must have been alive. . . .
>
> *Q.* When a woman has no assistance, may it not happen a child may be suffocated and smothered in the mess in which it is born with? *A.* I conceive it may very easily happen, without any intention of the kind. (*OB,* Oct. 1836: pp. 1017–20)

But suffocation was sometimes deliberate. A newborn baby was found inside a bundle in a coal cellar. A witness recalled that as "I removed the clothes, I found the head part with a coarse cloth over the face and neck. I looked down sideways, and said, 'Why the mouth is full of coarse cloth!'—it was three inches within the mouth." The hardened mass of cloth was found to have taken an exact cast of the mouth. However, as was frequently the case in infanticide, there had been no real autopsy. Under pressure from defense counsel, the medical expert found himself unable to exclude the possibility of death from some cause other than asphyxia (*OB,* Feb. 1817: pp. 155–57).

Forensic medical authorities recognized the importance of examining a putative mother for such signs of recent delivery as the appearance of the abdomen, breasts, and genitalia and the presence of lochia (Watson, 1842: pp. 281–84).

INSANITY

"Lactational insanity" or "puerperal mania," as it was also called, was a form of severe mental disturbance supposedly brought on by lactation. As such, this "temporary phrenzy" was occasionally invoked as an explanation for infanticide. In a typical case, the body of a dead infant was discovered two or three hours after its throat had been cut. John Rowland Gibson, the surgeon of Newgate Prison, testified at the trial of the accused mother:

> I visited her daily, and examined her. . . . I am of opinion that she is of weak intellect. . . . she could not tell me that two and two would

> make four, or that a quarter of a thing would be the fourth of it—I had some conversation with her about the case. . . . there is a sympathetic connection between the uterine organs and the brain—during conception and child-bearing, and afterwards, when giving milk, women are more susceptible of mental disturbance than at other periods—I think there is a great tendency to mental disturbance during delivery, and in the case of a person of weak intellect I think it might be increased. (*OB,* Nov. 1867: pp. 617–20)

John Johnstone, a respected nineteenth-century physician writing *On Madness* in 1800, accepted the concept of puerperal mania: "After parturition, delicate and irritable females are often liable to insanity, which at first shews itself in the form of delirium, but gradually degenerates into madness. This diseased state is probably occasioned by organic laesion, and its duration is proportional to the injury sustained" (pp. 16–17). John Conolly, a leading Victorian physician, agreed. "It is well known to medical men, that women are liable to temporary insanity after confinement" (1964: pp. 1 [intro.] and 424). William Hunter had earlier spoken of infanticide "committed under a phrenzy from despair,"[15] perhaps a more realistic explanation.

The Old Bailey trials for homicide of newborn infants make clear that, given the state of forensic medicine in the eighteenth and nineteenth centuries, it was very difficult to prove live birth from medical evidence. Aside from the problem of the legal definition of this state, there was the need to show beyond reasonable doubt that death had not occurred at a particular stage in the sequence of events which together constitute a delivery. Thus the objectivity of the lung flotation test gave it particular appeal. Although the procedure was called into question by some authorities almost as soon as it was derived, it was not discarded by all for more than two centuries. As one hard-pressed medical witness remarked, "It is our best test."

One is struck too with the way in which the savage statute of James I in time helped to stir public sympathy for the criminal acts of friendless, desperate, and socially helpless young women. When the latter came to trial, expert witnesses, often unsure themselves of the validity of their opinions, were likely to temper their conclusions, sometimes to the point of evident bias. There was obvious relief when the death penalty for this offense ceased to be mandatory.

15. 1783: p. 271. See also J. G. Smith, 1821: p. 310; Paris and Fonblanque, 1823: *3,* 129.

VII

Homicides of Children

HOMICIDES OF CHILDREN DIFFERED IN SEVERAL RESPECTS FROM THOSE of newborn infants and adults. In infanticide, homicide of the newborn, the concern of the mother was the concealment of a birth, and she acted as promptly as she was able. Adults who were murdered were most commonly victims of sudden passion; here again the lethal act was swift.[1] Child victims, however, were vulnerable to prolonged enmity or indifference, and their deaths by repeated beatings, starvation, or exposure were slow. Unlike threatened adults, endangered children found it difficult to speak for themselves, and if their murders came to light, it was when adults, finally alarmed, took action. It is probable that a great many of those responsible for the deaths of little children never were apprehended. According to Jackson (1982), in "the latter part of the nineteenth century, some 800 inquests were held each year in London on children under the age of two who were found dead in back alleys, privies, canals, and the river."

The ages of forty-five children whose alleged attackers came to trial at the Old Bailey appear in table 5. Beatings, starvation and exposure in some combination were responsible for at least thirty-two of the forty-five homicides. It was part of the task of the forensic medical expert to evaluate the relative importance of these and other lethal factors.

1. An exception were some homicidal deaths of the aged and helpless, destroyed in the same way as children.

CHILD LABORERS

Until well into the nineteenth century, young apprentices and other child laborers often, although not always, worked in conditions sufficiently unhealthy to be life-threatening. Under the Statute of Artificers and Apprentices of 1563, measures had been taken to regularize the training of apprentices, including young boys (5 Eliz. 1, c. 4). The Elizabethan Poor Law of 1601 stipulated that poor children were likely to get into trouble and must therefore be put to work; the statute permitted churchwardens and the overseers of workhouses to bind such children to masters to learn a trade (43 Eliz. 1, c. 2). The support of pauper children and orphans was the responsibility of the parish, which was naturally eager to rid itself of these financial burdens as promptly as possible. Furthermore, the children could be exploited with considerable profit to those parish overseers who were themselves employers. To stimulate the transfer of a child out of parish responsibility, a cash bonus was sometimes offered.

Poor parish children who were not apprenticed could be set to labor in workhouses in such jobs as picking oakum. Impoverished parents were free to exploit the labor of their own children in a family cottage industry such as hand-weaving. From Elizabeth's time until at least the early nineteenth century, such abuses continued and were taken for granted by a generally complacent public.

The results, as can be imagined, were appalling. Children, some of them only five years old, worked ten to twelve hours a day picking oakum. Hours for labor in the framework knitting trade were from five or six in the morning until ten at night. Food and housing were grossly inadequate, and sickness was widespread. Beatings were com-

Table 5. Ages of Victims in Child Homicide Trials at the Old Bailey

Age	No.	Age	No.
Under 3 months	6	6 years	1
3–6 months	7	8 years	1
7–11 months	6	11 years	2
1 year	5	12 years	2
2 years	5	15 years	1
3 years	1	Not stated	6
4 years	1	Total	45
5 years	1		

mon. Children were sometimes fastened to their machines. If a child died, it was easily replaced.

Public horror eventually was aroused, and in 1802 Sir Robert Peel successfully introduced the Health and Morals of Apprentices Act (42 Geo. 3, c. 73). Under this legislation, apprentices were not to work more than twelve hours a day. Not more than two were to sleep in a bed. Some provision was made for education and religious instruction. Mills and factories were to be inspected. Unfortunately, the act had little effect other than to call increased attention to a social evil. The Statute of Artificers and Apprentices Act was repealed in 1814 (54 Geo. 3, c. 96), and the state took no further responsibility for the protection and training of child laborers. New legislation passed in 1834 obliged poor children to work but protected only the interests of the employer. Decades were to pass before the situation improved significantly.[2]

There were eight trials at the Old Bailey between 1733 and 1829 for the murder of apprentices and other child laborers. Five of the victims were boys; three were girls. The oldest was fifteen, the youngest five years of age. In all, death, although perhaps coming finally as a result of particular violence, was the product of prolonged starvation, exposure, and beating.

> *John Bennet,* of Hammersmith, was indicted for the Murder of *George Main,* on the High-Seas, near *Sheerness,* in *England,* by beating him with a Stick call'd a Tiller, on the Head, Back, Shoulder, and Arms, and thereby giving him several Mortal Wounds on the 7th of *November,* of which Wounds he languish'd till the 2d of December following, and then dy'd, in the Hamlet of Hammersmith. He was a second time indicted on the Coroner's Inquisition for the said Murder.

The body was discovered hidden in the fishing boat. Autopsy showed head injuries and emaciation.

> Mr. *Duddle.* The *Dura Mater* was sound, but the *Pia Mater* much inflamed, and the Vessels much extended; the Vessels of the Brain were very turgid; the whole Substance of the Brain was much swell'd. Now the violent Concussion proceeding from the Blow, might so disturb and affect the Brain, as to occasion these Appearances, and so be the Cause of his Death.

The prisoner claimed that the boy had been fatally injured when he fell from the top of the fifteen-foot-high mast of the fishing boat. In spite

2. Bray, 1911: pp. 18–29; Payne, 1916: pp. 313–31; Hutchins and Harrison, 1926: pp. 2–6, 14–16, 20–25; Radbill, 1968: pp. 11–12; Longmate, 1974: p. 187.

of testimony by several witnesses as to his almost unbelievable cruelty, Bennet was found guilty of manslaughter (*OB,* Jan. 1733: pp. 30–34).

A hairdresser's apprentice, a boy of fifteen, died in the winter of cold and hunger. Said a neighbor, "I had a boiled mutton bone, I eat part of it, and flung the rest to the dog; the deceased came in and took it up, and seemed to eat it very savorily, as if he had ate nothing for a month." A surgeon at autopsy observed chilblains, ulceration of the feet, and emaciation (*OB,* Feb. 1776: pp. 180–84).

Probably most desperate of all was the situation of the "climbing boys" or chimney sweeps. In the nineteenth century heat for homes in London came from coal burned in sometimes numerous fireplaces. The flues of the latter were connected to chimneys. A chimney sweep, sent in to clean out the soot, could lose his way in these passages, which could be only nine inches square. Because of such dimensions, boys, and a few girls, were apprenticed at ages as young as five years to the master chimney sweeps. In this dangerous and terrifying trade the children were forced to work long hours and, it is said, were deliberately malnourished to retard their growth. Those who survived suffocation in a flue endured eyes chronically irritated by soot, scraped knees and elbows, and burns from the chimney fires they were expected to extinguish, and risked in later years the development of pulmonary tuberculosis or cancer of the scrotum as occupational diseases.

An account in the *Edinburgh Review* of 1819 summarized evidence presented in the House of Lords and House of Commons regarding the evils of this form of child labor. "*Little boys for small flues,* is a common phrase in the cards left at the door by itinerant chimney-sweepers." The children, it was reported, were often injured and sometimes crippled. They could be lost or trapped in a flue or chimney; if the master did not succeed in "smoking" them out by burning some straw below them, the chimney might have to be knocked down to release the child, earning him a beating. At night the sweeps slept in cellars, sometimes on piles of soot. Their clothing was ragged and scanty, and in cold weather chilblains were common. Work was heaviest in the winter months, much of it being done in the early hours of the morning before the fires were made up for the day.

A boy who managed to complete his apprenticeship would qualify as a journeyman and might eventually become a master sweep. Many of the latter turned their own children into climbing boys. Individuals who left the profession, ignorant, diseased, and perhaps crippled, were suited for little else and drifted into vagrancy and crime (Baldwin, 1819; Radbill, 1968: p. 12).

Statistics on the mortality of chimney sweeps seem to be scanty. Probably a good many deaths did not come to public attention. There were coroner's inquests into the deaths of four climbing boys in the City of London and Southwark between 1788 and 1829 (Forbes, 1978: pp. 20–21). In 1816 a man and his wife were tried at the Old Bailey for the murder of a five-year-old chimney sweep who worked for the male prisoner. Witnesses in a house where the chimneys were being cleaned had chanced to see the adult sweep beating the screaming child in the chimney with a long-handled brush. "I told him the child was not his own, or he would not use it so; he said it was nothing to me, and pulled him down by his legs, and dashed him down on the hearth stone. The child layed on its back, and received a violent blow on the back of its head by this fall. . . . The child was then put up the chimney; he lifted it up in his arms . . . and put the other boy after it. The other boy was about ten years old." Later the younger child was brought to the hospital with a contused forehead and mortification of the foot and leg secondary to a fractured femur. Because the infection was advanced, the limb was amputated; the child survived only a few minutes (*OB*, May 1816: pp. 263–64).

SUFFOCATION

Suffocation of a month-old baby was attempted by its mother. A neighbor in the same house, investigating noises, found the child under tightly tucked bedclothes with the sleeve of a shirt crammed into its mouth. She was lying on her face and moaning. Medical examination of the infant, still alive, at the police station disclosed emaciation and "lividity of the countenance, showing that air had been shut off for some period, and it was slightly convulsed. . . . it was quite impossible that it could have put the rag into its mouth itself."

The jury at the mother's trial for attempted murder apparently considered the possibility that she suffered from lactational insanity (see chapter 6). Asked the jurors, was the fact that she had not nursed the baby and her breasts were greatly distended "likely to affect her bodily health, or her mind?" No, said the medical witness, the period of accumulation was not long enough. The jury nevertheless recommended mercy because of the woman's recent confinement. She was sentenced to fifteen years' penal servitude (*OB*, July 1861: pp. 297–99).

OVERLYING

The suffocation of an infant by an older person lying on it has long been regarded as a possible cause of death. Certainly when one or more adults, not necessarily sober, slept in the same bed, or what passed for a bed, with a small baby, an accident could occur. Data on such deaths are not only relatively scanty but are necessarily incomplete and suspect. However, a report of the Registrar-General for all of England in the years 1852–56, disclosing a total of 5,464 violent deaths from all causes in children under one year of age, does ascribe 875 deaths to suffocation by bedclothes, 525 to overlying, 15 to murder, 14 to manslaughter, and 592 to infanticide by unspecified means (Nineteenth, 1858: pp. 167–75). Thomas Wakley, coroner of London at this time, on the other hand believed that overlying was rare. After a lengthy study of the circumstances of death in cases of alleged overlying he concluded in 1855 that "not one child out of two hundred who has been found dead in bed has lost its life in consequence of having been overlaid." Wakley thought that death was instead due to suffocation from bedclothes, pointing out that the largest numbers of deaths took place in the coldest months, the fewest in the warmest months (Inquests, 1855; Memoir, 1862). Modern pediatricians would also consider the sudden infant death syndrome (Hansen, 1979; Savitt, 1979).

Langer (1872, 1974) has conjectured that deliberate overlying was not uncommon in England and the Continent, to the extent that it and other forms of infanticide may in past centuries have been significant factors in population control.

Only one trial for infant homicide by overlying seems to have come to the Old Bailey before 1878. On Thursday, 20 May 1847, a surgeon visited a mother and her son, born the day before; the baby appeared to be quite well. When he saw the infant six hours later, it was lifeless, wrapped in a shawl and lying beside its mother in bed. The body "was then cold, the face was suffused, the nostrils dilated, there was a protrusion of the eye, the hands were clenched, the extremities of the fingers and the nails livid, and the legs drawn up towards the body." The surgeon became suspicious, perhaps in part because the mother was a prostitute, and went to the police.

At autopsy the examiners found congestion and extravasation in the lungs, liver, and left side of the brain. The other viscera appeared to be healthy. It was concluded that death was due to suffocation. Admittedly this surgeon had never before seen an allegedly overlain baby. Criminal intent on the part of the mother was not proved, and she was acquitted (*OB,* June 1847: pp. 346–59).

TRAUMA VERSUS DISEASE

When a young homicide victim had also suffered from a major illness, it was sometimes difficult to answer the all important question: What was the primary cause of death? In 1828 a little girl, Frances Colpit, five or six years old and allegedly in good health, was taken from St. Martin's Workhouse and "articled as an apprentice to Esther Hibner, Sen., of Platt's-terrace, to learn the business of a tambour-worker, she engaging to provide her with board, lodging, and all other necessaries."[3] Some months later the parish overseer visited Mrs. Hibner's house to inspect the children who had been placed there. Six were so ill that they were removed. Little Frances, cut, bruised, and emaciated, later died.

On the witness stand at Esther Hibner's trial for murder, another apprentice told how Frances daily had been

> called up to work between three and four o'clock, and continued to work till between ten and eleven at night, from Michaelmas till the time she went away; she used to have a slice of dry bread, and a cup of milk and water at breakfast time; she had nothing else in the course of the day, and no other meal till the next morning—she had her breakfast at half-past eight o'clock, and was allowed five minutes to eat in. . . . the son had some pigs; the man who minded them used to have the wash [kitchen swill] from the tavern, and when that has been brought for the dog I have seen Colpit, Foster and Howse take and eat it. . . . if we had not done our work mistress used to keep us without victuals, and she used to give us a good flogging before we went to bed.

At the child's autopsy her toes were found to be severely mortified. She was very emaciated and the abdomen was inflamed. Death, however, was ascribed to tuberculous abscesses of the lung. "I think dipping her head two or three times into a pail of water very likely to bring the tubercles into action."

3. A tambour was a circular frame on which cloth was stretched for embroidery.

Ester Hibner was condemned to the gallows (*OB,* April 1829: pp. 350–55).

ORGANIZED CHILD HOMICIDE

A shocking number of child deaths resulted from the corruption of two supposedly benevolent social institutions. One of these was the practice of employing women to care in their homes for abandoned or destitute infants and small children. At its best, a foster home could provide kindly nurture, food, shelter, and clothing for one or more babies, perhaps in a much better environment than they had previously experienced. At the other extreme was a purely commercial venture whose operators charged a parent or a parish as much in fees as the traffic would bear, spent as little as possible on the children, and callously waited for or even expedited the deaths of their helpless charges. Charles Dickens paints the grim scene in more than one of his novels.

Orphans, the children of paupers, and babies abandoned by their parents became, as earlier stated, the responsibility of the parish in which they were born. The parishioners had little sympathy for the offspring, often illegitimate, of social failures and outcasts, resented paying for the support of the children, and looked for the cheapest solution. Women made a business of engaging for a flat fee to look after these parish charges. If the infants did not survive for long, both the "killing nurses" or "angel makers," as they were sometimes known, and the parish overseers stood to gain. A domicile where numerous small children were placed for this kind of care was known as a "baby farm."[4] Radbill tells us that of the illegitimate babies "put out to nurse" in London in the 1800s, 80 percent perished, a startling figure even when one allows for the high infant mortality rates still prevailing in the nineteenth century.[5]

As the result of a baby-farming scandal in September 1870, Margaret Waters, aged thirty-five, and her sister, Sarah Ellis, aged twenty-eight, were tried for the murder of John Walter Cowen, aged four weeks. During the trial it developed that one Robert Cowen, learning

4. The term was familiar enough for W. S. Gilbert to use it in "Buttercup's Song," act 2, of *H.M.S. Pinafore,* written in 1878.

5. Radbill, 1968: p. 7; 1974: p. 243. See also Langer, 1972: p. 97; 1974: p. 360; Wrightson, 1975: p. 16; Sauer, 1978: p. 87.

that his unmarried daughter was pregnant, had responded to an advertisement in *Lloyd's Weekly Newspaper* for 1 May 1870:

> Adoption.—A respectable couple desire the entire charge of a child to bring up as their own. They are in a position to offer every comfort. Premium required, 4*l*. Letter only. Mrs. Willis, P.O., Southampton Street, Camberwell.

The next day an answer to Cowen's inquiry arrived in the post:

> Sir, In reply to your letter, beg to say we are not willing to give our address. In taking a child we wish to do so entirely, never to be claimed. We have been married many years, but are without family, and have determined upon bringing a little one up as our own. My constant care shall be for the child, and everything which will be for the child's comfort shall be strictly studied. Should you think more of this, and will write saying where and when I can see you and how I shall know you, we shall feel obliged. We have had several letters, so are anxious to decide which child we shall take.
>
> Yours respectfully, M. Willis.

Later "M. Willis," actually Margaret Waters, and Sarah Ellis were identified in court by a clerk in the advertising department of the newspaper as the persons who had placed that advertisement and several others like it between January 1869 and June 1870—"we have had advertisements of the same sort spread over a number of years, from persons professing to undertake the care of children . . . a great many." A police sergeant identified the handwriting in the manuscript of the 1 May advertisement as that of Waters, and twenty-seven other such documents were stated to be in her hand or that of Ellis.

Margaret Waters and Robert Cowen met by arrangement at Brixton Railway Station on 3 May. She told him that her husband was with a ship-building firm and that they had been married thirteen years but had no children. Cowen informed Waters that his daughter was not married and that her baby would be born in about two weeks at the house of a midwife, Mrs. Castle. The birth occurred on 14 May. Cowen thereupon himself placed an advertisement, "M. Willis" having refused to divulge her address, to notify her of the birth of a healthy son. Eventually it was arranged that Waters would pick up the infant at Walworth Road Station on the evening of 7 June, which she did. Three days later Walters called on Cowen, reporting that she and her husband were delighted with the baby and that she was busy making clothes for it. After many protestations, she accepted £2 from Cowen.

By the beginning of June the police had become suspicious. A Sergeant Relf was instructed to watch the house of Mrs. Castle, the midwife.[6] Under the name of J. Martin, Sergeant Relf responded to an advertisement in *Lloyd's Weekly Newspaper* for 5 June which read like that seen by Mr. Cowen: "A good home, with a mother's love and care, is offered," etc. This notice ended with the instruction, "Apply by letter only to Mrs. Oliver, P.O. Gore Place, Brixton." Relf answered on 8 and 9 June with letters alleging his interest, and on the latter date met "Mrs. Oliver"—the prisoner Ellis—at Camberwell New Road Railway Station. He identified himself as J. Martin. She acknowledged the letter she had addressed to him under that name, a missive along the same lines as that received by Cowen. She told Relf that her husband was a "house decorator and painter, in a large way of business."

The detective promised to bring Ellis a child the next night and to pay her £5. By prearrangement, Cowen was concealed nearby so that he could identify her. Relf shadowed Ellis to her house, thereby discovering its location.

The next morning, 10 June, the police sergeant, Cowen, and Mrs. Guerra, the latter's housekeeper, went to Ellis's house. Cowen stayed outside, while Relf and Mrs. Guerra knocked at the door, which

> was opened by Mrs. Ellis—the house was a very nice house outside, but there was hardly any furniture in it, and it smelt very offensively—there were six rooms. . . . when Ellis opened the door, I said "Does Mrs. Willis live here?"—she said "No" I said "Do you take children in here to adopt?" she said "No, what put that in your head?"—I said "Is Miss Cowen's child here?"—she said "No, but I know where it is; will you step in and wait?"—I said "No, I shall not leave you a second till Miss Cowen's child is produced"—she then took us into the front room on the ground floor, and called out "Margaret, bring up Miss Cowen's child," and a child was brought up by the prisoner Waters; it was very emaciated, and very dirty, in fact, filthy—it was wrapped up in some old clothes, and was a mere skeleton, mere skin and bone—it was quite quiet, and did not appear to have power to cry, or make any noise.

It must be recalled that this was less than three days after a supposedly healthy twenty-four-day-old baby had been turned over to the Waters woman. Relf's testimony continued.

6. She may have specialized both in accepting unmarried women for delivery in her home and in informing the baby farmers of prospective clients.

> Mrs. Guerra said "You have been starving this child to death"—Waters said that the child had been ill, and had been attended by Dr. Harris; that it had plenty of milk, which her milk bills would show—I then asked her if she had got any more children in the house, and she said "A few"—I said "I should like to see them"—she said I could, and I went downstairs into the front kitchen; when I first went in I saw nothing, but I thought I could see something that looked like the shape of a head under some black clothes on a sofa—at last I removed some clothing from the sofa, and there laid five infants, all huddled up together. . . . all five lay in the same direction—they all had some clothing on, infants' clothes, and very dirty indeed, saturated with wet, and smelt very offensively—I did not see any appearance of food about—two of the infants appeared to me to be dying. . . . Waters said she did not know who the parents were—I said "Are those some more by adoption?"—she said "Yes"—I then said in the presence of Ellis, "Have you any more?"—she said "Yes, a few; there are some older ones in the yard"—I went into the back yard, and there found five more; they appeared in better condition, one boy was a very fine child—I said to Waters "These children look better, how do you account for that?"—she said "We have [are paid] so much a week with these"—I then left the house, and fetched Dr. Puckle, the medical officer of the parish.

About two hours later the police sergeant, the doctor, and Cowen returned to the house. The Cowen baby "looked like a shrivelled up monkey." Waters said that

> the child had been ill, and she had had Dr. Harris to attend to it; and also that she was going to put it out to wet-nurse that day—I then went downstairs, I found the five infants still there—they had all got nice clean clothes on then, and were laid in rows on the sofa, and feeding bottles by their sides, and teats in their mouths. . . . they were all in this quiet state, apparently asleep; I mean they appeared to be void of any feeling, in a state of torpor, unconscious, in a state of stupor. . . . I observed this bottle (*produced*) on the table, with the cork out and lying by it—this was in the kitchen where the infants were—I smelt it and thought it was laudanum—Dr. Puckle also smelt it.

It developed that a sixth unconscious baby was Ellis's.

The Cowen baby was turned over to a wet nurse. The nine children, the Ellis child excepted, were removed first to Police Court and then to Lambeth Workhouse, although not until Monday, 13 June. On that day also, Ellis and Waters were taken into custody.

At the police station Mrs. Waters was unable to identify any except the Ellis and Cowen infants. The police therefore numbered them 1,

2, 3, 4, 5, 6, 7, 8, and 9. The sergeant asked Waters, "How long have you been in this business?"—she said "About four years"—I said "How many have you had in that time?"—she said "About forty"—Ellis said "Oh, more than forty"—Waters said "Oh no, say forty."

When the two prisoners were searched, over £11 and seventy-nine pawnbrokers' tickets were found among their possessions. The articles that had been pawned, for a total of £7 or £8, were soiled children's clothing and numerous pieces of furniture. It was learned from a written statement found in the prisoners' house that it had been rented by Waters under the name of Margaret Blackburn.

Dr. George Puckle, Medical Officer of Health for Lambeth, testified that he had first examined the Cowen baby:

> the body of the child was very much emaciated, extremely wasted, the bones almost coming through the skin—it was a miserably wasted child, no flesh hardly on the bones . . . and it had that aged appearance in the face which made it difficult to form an opinion of its age. . . . it was in a thoroughly insensible state; the eyes were closed, the limbs hung down, and it appeared in a very profound stupor—I raised the eyelids, and found the pupils very much contracted, not in a natural state. . . . my opinion is that the child was in a state of narcotism, arising from the administration of some narcotic poison—laudanum would be the very thing that I should suppose had been administered. . . . I asked Waters about the child having been ill—she said it had suffered from diarrhea and from thrush—I saw that it had suffered from thrush.

Waters denied having administered sleeping medicine or soothing syrup.

The Cowen baby died on 24 June, in Puckle's opinion "of a combined cause, atrophy, or extreme wasting, with exhaustion and congestion of the brain. . . . in my judgment death arose from want of suitable food sufficiently early, and also from the improper administration of a narcotic."

The doctor testified that four of the other babies had also died. Their autopsies indicated that "congestion of the brain formed a very important part of the cause of death of these four infants." As to the small bottle found beside the unconscious children in the kitchen, Puckle was convinced that the few drops it still contained were laudanum.

Dr. Henry Bullen, a surgeon and the Medical Officer of the Lambeth Workhouse, described the nine children brought there from the police station on 13 June. Two were judged to be two or three years old, the others from three weeks to eighteen months in age. Of the nine, the three oldest were in good health and "were subsequently claimed and removed." Numbers 4 and 5 were fast recovering. Numbers 6, 7, 8, and 9, from three months to three weeks old, had died. All had shown great emaciation and a torpid, inanimate condition, the latter caused, Bullen believed, by "some soporific drug." He had had, he said, considerable experience with neglected, emaciated children who were brought to the workhouse. If a suitable wet nurse could not be found, it was, he conceded, difficult to "bring them up by hand," that is, by artifical feeding.

> MR. SERJEANT BALLANTINE *proposed to call a witness in order to prove the finding under a railway arch [of] the body of an infant, upon which were articles of clothing and papers that would be traced to one of the prisoners. The evidence was tendered for the purpose of shewing a systematic reception by the prisoners of infants, and the disposition of their bodies after death, so as to lead to the inference that in the case of John Walter Cowen, they contemplated his death.* THE LORD CHIEF BARON *was of opinion that such evidence was wholly inadmissible, being quite unconnected with the cause of the death of the child in question.*

Shortly afterward, the Lord Chief Baron decided that there was no evidence against Ellis "and directed the Jury to find a verdict of NOT Guilty as to her." She was set free. Waters was found guilty and sentenced to death. By order of the court, a reward of £20 was given to Sergeant Relf (*OB,* Sept. 1870: pp. 539–71).

The burial societies were another threatening social institution. These may be classed with foster homes in that, while both might be valuable to society, they also could constitute a serious hazard for babies and small children. The burial clubs provided an appalling opportunity for financial gain to the parents of children who perished after having been enrolled.

The premium for a child's membership was about £1. The burial club allowed a payment to the parents of £3 to £5 when a child died. Since the cost of a funeral was from £1 to £1 10s., the "profit" was considerable, particularly when a child had been enrolled in not one but several clubs. Ryan tells of a minister in the Manchester area who had been repeatedly shocked to hear it said of a baby, "'Aye, aye, that child will not live; IT IS IN THE BURIAL CLUB.'" One Manchester parent insured his child in nineteen of the societies. It was learned that another youngster, discovered to have been deliberately starved to death, "*had been entered in at least ten burial* clubs, and the parents had six other children who only lived from nine to eighteen months respectively. They had received twenty pounds, from several burial clubs, for *one of these children.*"

Although at the trial of these parents evidence was presented of their systematic starvation of the first-mentioned child, the jury reached an inconclusive verdict. Proof of the deliberate homicide was felt insufficient for conviction. Thereupon the parents, discharged from the court, enforced payment from *ten* burial clubs, collecting £34 3*s*.[7]

7. Ryan, 1862: pp. 20–24; Havard, 1960: pp. 51–53, 59–60; Radbill, 1968: p. 7; Sauer, 1978: pp. 87–88.

VIII

Poisoning

IN FEBRUARY OF THE YEAR 1532 JOHN FISHER, BISHOP OF ROCHESTER, was residing with a large household at his mansion in Lambeth Marsh. One day it chanced that a pot filled with yeast and other ingredients for making porridge stood in the kitchen. The cook, one Richard Roose, chose to add to the mixture "a certain venym or pyson." His reason we do not know.[1] The porridge was served to the residents of the household and what was left was given, as was the custom, to hungry citizens waiting at the door. Before long, seventeen members of the household were desperately ill and one of them, Benett Curwen, gentleman, had died. These were not all. Several of the "pore people which resorted to the sayde Bysshops place and were there charytably fedde with the remaynes of the saide porrage and other vytayles [victuals], were in lyke wyse infected, and one pore Woman of them, that is to saye, Alice Trppyn wydowe is also thereof nowe deceased."

Parliament reacted to this murderous deed by passing a special statute (22 Hen. 8, c. 9), the preamble to which expressed horror at homicide and particularly at poisoning, "which in this Realme hytherto our Lorde be thanked hath been moste rare and seldom commytted or practysed." The giving of poison Parliament now adjudged to constitute high treason. Richard Roose and others convicted of the

1. It has been suggested (Mullinger, 1908) that this was an attempted assassination of the bishop, who had incurred the wrath of Anne Boleyn because he opposed the divorce of Henry VIII from Katherine of Aragon.

crime were to lose their benefit of clergy[2] and to be boiled to death (Statutes, 1817: *3*, 326). Roose perished at Smithfield, as did three or four others convicted of poisoning, before the act was repealed in 1547 (1 Edw. 6, c. 12; Stephen, 1883: 1, 476–77; 3, 44–45).

Homicidal poisoning was in several respects an unusual crime. Under the law, it was always regarded as murder, never as manslaughter, since the offense was considered to have been deliberate and premeditated; the poisoner intended to kill (Glaister, 1954: p. 12; Adelson, 1974: p. 725). In a trial for poisoning, the burden of proof was on the prosecution, and the accused might not attempt to show that he or she was not guilty. Of all murderers, the poisoner was and is regarded as the most difficult to convict. If clever, he finds full opportunity to plan carefully, to select the time and place, and to cover his tracks. Poisoning is commonly a domestic crime, to be perpetrated secretly against an unsuspecting victim. The choice of a poison depends largely, as Adelson states, on the ease with which it can be obtained and on the poisoner's impression, not always correct, of how the poison will act (1974: p. 729). After the offense is committed, external signs are usually few. Because poisoning is relatively uncommon, it is a crime with which the authorities have little familiarity (Glaister, 1954: pp. 11–15; 1960: pp. 82–83).

In past centuries medical men called to the scene of a deliberate poisoning might well fail to grasp what had happened. A careful poisoner would leave no empty bottle, no food laced with arsenic, no lingering odor of laudanum. Witnesses might tell of a rapid or a lingering death. Common symptoms—failing heart, respiratory distress, abdominal pain, unconsciousness—after all were characteristic of many kinds of illness. Fatal poisoning from spoiled food was a not uncommon accident. There was no wound or bruise, no knife or club, and the victim most often had died at home in the bosom of his family.

Probably no other kind of homicide offered greater challenge to the alert medical practitioner. His ability to observe and interpret all he saw, including minute details, to evaluate and diagnose, needed to be at its most acute. A healthy measure of suspicion was valuable. Obviously a thorough post-mortem examination would be essential. Even so, the surgeon would be handicapped by the fact that some poisons were eliminated from the body before death. And, of course, toxicology and pathology were scarcely past their infancy. The first

2. Exemption from secular courts and capital punishment was granted originally only to the clergy, later to anyone connected with the Church, and finally to "clerks," that is, to anyone who could read.

reliable and specific test for a poison, arsenic, was not to be discovered until 1836. How did the physician or surgeon cope? There can be little doubt that a good many homicidal poisonings went undetected or unproven. Even if a medical man's suspicions were stirred, what steps would he take? What knowledge was there to assist him?

An early British investigator of the actions of poisons was Richard Mead, who in 1702 wrote what appears to be the first book in English on the subject. He discussed the venom of the viper, tarantula, and mad dog, poisonous minerals (mercury and arsenic compounds), poisonous plants (*Cicuta,* the water hemlock, and aconite, or monkshood), opium, and "venomous exhalations," by which term he meant fumes from swamps—the *mephites,* which supposedly caused malaria—and from mines, caves, and pits. Also included were the human exhalations by which certain diseases were spread, and poisonous springs. Mead administered toxic minerals to experimental animals and then autopsied their bodies (1702). Similar investigations were conducted early in the nineteenth century by the distinguished surgeon Sir Benjamin Brodie, who described the actions of eleven different poisons in test animals and also wrote about his experiments with various methods for the resuscitation of victims of poison (1811, 1812).

A few years later, in a fascinating little volume entitled *An Essay into the Operation of Poisonous Agents upon the Living Body,* John Morgan and Thomas Addison, surgeon and physician, respectively, of Guy's Hospital,[3] related their experiments on the effects of various poisons in animals.[4] Through ingenious experiments they reached the conclusion that "all poisons, and perhaps, indeed, all agents influence the brain and general system, through an impression made upon the sentient extremities of the nerves, and not by absorption and direct application to the brain" (1829: p. 90). Although these investigators interpreted their data incorrectly, their studies represent important advances in toxicology.

But the reports of Mead, Brodie, and Morgan and Addison did not include a discussion of how the new findings might be applied to forensic medicine, at that time still an unfamiliar field. It is true that Samuel Farr's early but not original *Elements of Medical Jurisprudence*

3. Addison (1793–1860) is best known for his description of the disease of the suprarenal glands which bears his name. Actually he had confused this malady with pernicious anemia (Mettler, 1947: pp. 434–35).

4. Contrary to Garrison (1929: p. 422), theirs is not "the first book in English on the action of poisons on the living body," being antedated by Mead's volume of 1702.

had advocated in cases of suspected human poisoning the feeding of the victim's dried stomach contents "to other animals, such as fowls, dogs, &c. which if it causes their death, or violent vomiting, it is a proof inter aliae, that poison made a part of its contents" (1819: p. 53).

Robert Christison's *A Treatise on Poisons,* appearing in 1829, was the first comprehensive presentation in English on the subject. Christison, a former student of Orfila, the great Spanish student of toxicology, and deeply influenced by him, had been appointed to the Chair of Medical Jurisprudence at the University of Edinburgh in 1822, when he was not yet twenty-four. The materials accumulated for his lectures became the *Treatise* (Parker, 1973: pp. v–vii). In this lengthy work—the first edition ran to 698 pages (1829a)—he divided toxic materials into three classes: irritant poisons (inorganic and some animal and vegetable compounds); narcotic poisons (including not only opium, its derivatives, and *Hyoscyamus, Lactuca,* and *Solanum,* but also hydrocyanic acid and poisonous gases); and narcotico-acrid poisons (various plant substances and alcohol). Christison stirred in the brilliant young William Brooke O'Shaughnessy (1809–89), an Edinburgh medical graduate, an interest in forensic chemistry which was to lead him to numerous contributions in that field (Gorman, 1984).

Alfred Swaine Taylor's volume *On Poisons,* which succeeded Christison's classic in 1848 and ultimately replaced it, made use of the same classification. As would be expected, Taylor's treatise dealt thoroughly and in detail with toxicology as it was then understood, citing numerous cases with references from the British, Continental, and American scientific literature. Constant attention was given to the sources, availability, and even cost of a poison, to the symptoms it produced, to differentiation of such symptoms from those of certain diseases, to the best available methods for attempting the identification of a poison, and to rules to be observed in investigating cases of poisoning. There can be no doubt of Taylor's influence, both on textbooks, which gave increasing attention to the medicolegal aspects of toxicology, and on the practice of forensic medicine. More than 40 percent of the 1877 edition of Woodman and Tidy's *Forensic Medicine and Toxicology* was devoted to poisoning.

Most fatal cases of poisoning were accidental, a smaller number were suicidal, and fewest of all were homicidal. Hatrick found that of each eleven thousand deaths from all causes in London in 1859, only one was due to poison (1862). But such estimates were based on returns supplied by coroners, a source of information deprecated by the statistician William Farr. Said he: "It was stated before a Committee of the House of Commons in 1851, that the constabulary of Staffordshire were instructed not to furnish 'notices' of deaths to the coroners except when crime was *suspected*. And the coroners were informed, that if they held inquests in such cases their fees would be disallowed. Under these circumstances Palmer committed several murders." Commenting on the reports supplied by coroners to the Registrar General of England and Wales for his annual reports, Farr stated that in the five years 1852–56 there was a yearly average of 13,711 violent deaths. Among these

> 401 persons died *annually* of poisoning, and in nearly 113 cases the poison is not specified. Opium is the principal specified poison. . . . 34 persons were killed annually by prussic acid. . . . Arsenic stands next, and to it 27 deaths are referred. The salts of lead kill 23 persons annually, the salts of mercury kill 10, oxalic acid kills 13, sulphuric acid (oil of vitriol) kills 15 persons annually. The deaths from these poisons are understated, as the 113 deaths from unspecified poisons are chiefly caused by them, and in some cases the poisoning is not discovered, and the death is erroneously ascribed to disease. (1885: pp. 292 *f.*, 294)

Some years earlier, a Parliamentary report, *Returns from the Coroners of England and Wales, of all Inquisitions held by them during the years 1837 and 1838, in cases where death was found, by Verdict of Jury, to have been caused by Poisoning,* was summarized in the *Lancet* (Statistics, 1839). Part of this information appears in table 6.

It appears that the majority of the 540 fatal poisonings listed in the table were the result of accidents, intoxication, or lunacy. At least forty-eight more were from overdoses administered by an adult to a child or children. An additional twenty-seven fatalities were suicidal, and at least five were caused by abortifacients. Only seven—five by arsenic and two by laudanum—of the 504 poisonings, or 0.014 percent were recognized as homicidal.[5]

Among Old Bailey trials in 1739–1878, eighty-three for poisoning were encountered. The distribution of these cases by decade is indicated in table 7. Note the clustering of sixty-three of the trials in 1839–78; the reasons for this phenomenon are uncertain. Of the eighty-three cases, forty-nine involved charges of homicide and thirty-one of attempted homicide. Two poisoning cases were related to robberies

5. More than a century later, of 3,118 fatal poisonings investigated in Cuyahoga County, Ohio, in 1943–71, only 15, or 0.005 percent, were homicides, testimony to the continuing rarity of murder by poison (Adelson, 1974: p. 728).

Table 6. Poison Deaths in England and Wales, 1837–1838

185	Opium, laudanum, syrup of poppies, elixir of paregoric, "infant's mixture," morphine acetate	2	"Medicine," "decoction"
184	Arsenic	2	Morrison's pills, "Hierapicra" (*hiera picra*)
32	Vitriol (sulfuric acid)	1	Cough syrup
31	Prussic (hydrocyanic) acid, oil of almonds	1	Hellebore
19	Oxalic acid	1	Potassium bichromate
14	Unspecified poisons	1	Silver nitrate (as percussion caps)
14	Corrosive sublimate, mercury	1	Castor oil seeds
12	Godfrey's cordial	1	Rum
5	Nux vomica, strychnine	1	Lead extract
4	Fungus	1	Prussic acid and arsenic
3	Vegetable poison	1	Prussic acid and laudanum
2	Tartar emetic	1	Arsenious acid
2	"Mixture for vermin"	1	Wolfsbane (aconite)
2	Aqua fortis (nitric acid)	1	Ferrous sulfate
2	Carburetted hydrogen gas (methane)	1	Monkshood
2	Belladonna or deadly nightshade	1	Savine
2	"Black ashes for washing" (potash)	1	Infusion of hemlock
		1	Muriate of tin (stannic chloride)
		1	Cantharides
		1	Laudanum and aqua fortis
		1	Nitrous acid and aloes
		1	Cayenne pepper
		1	Turpeth mineral (turbith)
	Total	540	

Source: Statistics of poisoning in England. *Lancet* 1 (1839):597–99.

Table 7. Old Bailey Poisoning Cases by Decade

1739–48	1	1809–18	2
1749–58	1	1819–28	4
1759–68	1	1829–38	7
1769–78	2	1839–48	23
1779–88	0	1849–58	17
1789–98	0	1859–68	7
1799–08	2	1869–78	16
		Total	83

Table 8. Old Bailey Trials for Poisoning, 1739–1878: Poisons Used

Poison	Homicide	Attempted homicide	Other	Total	Poison	Homicide	Attempted homicide	Other	Total
Potassium sulfate	2[a]			2	Strychnine	3			3
Unnamed abortifacient		1[a]		1	*Cocculus indicus*			1[b]	1
Arsenic	12	7		19	Opium, morphia		1		1
Corrosive sublimate	2	1		3	Laudanum	5	4		9
Ammoniated mercury		3		3	Foxglove	1			1
Lead acetate	2	1		3	Belladonna	1	1		2
Tartar emetic		1		1	Hydrocyanic acid	4	1		5
Tartaric acid	1			1	Oxalic acid	1	5		6
Vitriol	1	2		3	Cantharides	1	1		2
Aqua fortis	1	1		2	Alcohol	5			5
Morrison's pills	1			1	Chloral		1		1
Savin	1[a]			1	Chloroform			2[c]	2
Lobelia	2			2	Not identified	3			3
					Total	49	31	3	83

[a] Attempted abortion.
[b] River poisoning.
[c] Robbery.

and one to poisoning a river. Not included in this count were the additional cases of child murder in which opium derivatives probably played a role (see chapter 7). At least twenty-five different toxic substances were involved in the Old Bailey cases (table 8).[6]

POTASSIUM SULFATE

Potassium sulfate in a dose of one drachm (one-eighth of an ounce) was sometimes prescribed as a mild purgative, being regarded as relatively innocuous. But, like many other substances, it was lethal when taken in sufficiently large quantity.

In 1843 a husband gave his wife over a period of about two weeks a total of half a pound of potassium sulfate in divided doses in order to induce an abortion. She became very ill, vomited, and died in a few hours. Autopsy revealed that the wife was not pregnant. Death was reported due to a ruptured cerebral blood vessel. The stomach and intestines were highly inflamed; this condition, it was vaguely suggested, might have caused apoplexy. The husband was found not guilty (*OB,* Oct. 1843: pp. 1025–29).

Only a few years later a medical man showed what skill and knowledge could accomplish in a poisoning case. Once again potassium sulfate had been administered as an abortifacient. Dr. Henry Letheby determined by chemical analysis that there were seventy-four grains (4.795 grams) of the substance in two teacups found at the scene of the poisoning. He demonstrated more of the chemical in a residue of vomitus on the carpet, estimating that the victim probably received about an ounce and a half (42.5 grams), which he said would be a fatal dose. The woman who died was also found on post-mortem examination not to be pregnant (*OB,* Oct. 1856: pp. 963–66).

ARSENIC

In February 1692 Edward Francis, a "blackamoor" servant, was tried in the City of London for treasonably murdering his mistress, Jane Dymock.[7] Her husband, Thomas Dymock, was the Keeper of the

6. The substances in table 8 have been classified as in the contemporary textbook of Woodman and Tidy (1877: pp. x–xii).

7. The charge was petty treason, the killing of a person to whom allegiance was owed, as to a master or mistress by a servant or to a husband by a wife.

Lions at the Tower of London, where there was at that time a small menagerie. In the summer of 1690 the servant bought a sixpenny parcel of ratsbane, or arsenic, from a ratcatcher, putting some in milk that was then served to his master. Thomas Dymock soon was ill indeed. At intervals over the next year and a half, more arsenic was administered to him and Mistress Dymock. Thomas became desperately sick and his wife Jane died.

After several months, the master having remarried, Francis used the poison again, this time in a skillet of water gruel. Soon the second wife became acutely ill, as did a servant and Dymock's daughter Elizabeth, who later recalled that when she "tooke the water grewell and did eate it, it seemed to be Hott and Burning in my Mouth," a symptom characteristic of arsenic poisoning. An additional victim was "the Catt by chance eating what was left in the Porringer of the Grewell"; it died at once. Edward Francis, by this time an obvious suspect, "confest that he did it with a Design to poyson this Examinant [Thomas Dymock] & be master himself." His lack of subtlety suggests a simple, perhaps even an unbalanced, mind. He was acquitted (Examination, 1692; City, 1692).

Arsenic, familiar since the Middle Ages, exists in various forms. The common variety, arsenous oxide, or white arsenic, looks like sugar or flour, has little taste, is not very soluble in water, and is highly poisonous. In past centuries it was cheap and easily available, being frequently employed not only as a rodent poison but also as an insecticide, sheep dip, preservative of feed grain, and so on. Copper arsenite, Scheele's green, was used as a pigment in wallpaper, toys, and fabrics, and sometimes as a color for candy and blancmange (Guy and Ferrier, 1875: p. 450; Campbell, 1965). Arsenic not only is widely distributed in nature but occurs normally in trace amounts in the human body, a fact which was to complicate expert testimony on more than one occasion. Another forensic medical difficulty was that the symptoms of arsenic poisoning were known to resemble those of cholera, prevalent on occasion in the nineteenth century (Taylor, 1848: pp. 51, 54).

Of the nineteen trials for arsenic poisoning at the Old Bailey up to 1878, nine occurred between 1752 and 1844, with eight more in the short span from May 1846 to August 1850. This last outbreak may have spurred Parliament to pass in 1850 a bill to regulate the sale of the substance (14 Vict., c. 14). But instances of arsenic poisoning continued.

Until the advent of reliable analytic tests, evidence in the prosecution of a charge of murder by poison was likely to be both circumstantial and hard to come by. The expert medical witness on whom so much depended was too often severely handicapped by inexperience in toxicology. Suspicion was not enough. Proof was needed that death was indeed due to a toxic agent rather than, say, to disease, that a particular poison had been administered in a lethal dose, and that the accused was responsible. An example of a trial in which these elements were lacking to an extent shocking by modern standards was that of Richard Weston in 1615 for the fatal poisoning of Sir Thomas Overbury.

This notorious and complex affair involved not only commoners but highly placed members of the nobility and the professions, linked in personal and political intrigue.[8] At the center were what were alleged to be repeated attempts to poison Overbury during the summer of 1613 while he was a prisoner in the Tower. Richard Weston, the accused, was Under Keeper to the Lieutenant of the Tower. Brought to trial, Weston at first refused to plead, even under threat of the torture *peine forte et dure*. But four days later he changed his mind. Standing again at the bar and asked once more how he answered to the indictment, he responded, "By God and by my country," that is, not guilty. Weston was charged with having given Overbury realgar (arsenic disulfide, red arsenic, used in fireworks and as a pigment) on 9 May, white arsenic in June, tarts containing mercury sublimate on 10 July, and a clyster or enema of the same substance on 14 September, when Overbury had died. During all these months he had received medical attention.

A coroner's jury had viewed the body on the day of death, finding the corpse emaciated and marked with ulcers, blisters, and other sores. Since one Paul de Lobell, an apothecary,[9] had testified that when he had bathed the ailing Overbury on 3 July his body "was exceeding fair and clear" and since poisons were thought to cause blisters and decay,[10] the lesions discovered on Overbury's corpse were regarded as evidence of poisoning. However, there was no autopsy.

Lord Chief Justice Sir Edward Coke, noted jurist and legal historian, had already prepared the prosecution's case for presentation by

8. For details, Beatrice White's *A Cast of Ravens* (1965) is recommended.

9. He was the son of Matthias de Lobell, or de l'Obel (1538–1616), born in Lille, who practiced medicine in Holland and later in London, where he was physician and botanist to James I. For the father is named the familiar flower *Lobelia*.

10. An error still entertained in the nineteenth century (Pettigrew, 1818).

the Queen's Attorney. Now Coke, as was permitted under the rules of the day, served also as one of Weston's judges. Notable was his instruction to the jury: "albeit the poisoning in the indictment be said to be with rosalgar, white arsenic, and mercury sublimate, yet the jury are not to expect precise proof on that point" (quoted by deFord, 1960: p. 60), nor was any supplied. Coke's explanation for this extraordinary statement was that no one had *seen* Weston preparing the poisonous food and drink (Parry, 1925: p. 221). Actually, the evidence for much of what was charged against Weston was in any case circumstantial or hearsay, and proof of his guilt was scanty. Nevertheless he was found guilty of murder and went to the gallows on 25 October 1615. Many honest lawyers recoiled at the illegalities of the proceedings.[11]

In the next century and a half, proof of poisoning made little if any progress. Certain symptoms and allegedly distinctive post-mortem stigmata, notably rapid putrefaction, continued to be regarded as indicative that a poison (other than arsenic) had caused death. The trial of Mary Blandy in 1752 at Oxford is said to be the first, or one of the first, in which chemical tests for arsenic were accepted as evidence (Glaister, 1960: Mant, 1977). This woman was charged with the murder of her father. Briefly, the circumstances preceding the father's death were that a Captain Cranstoun, a married man who had heard that Mary was to inherit £10,000, convinced her to agree to marry him. The girl's father suspected and disliked Cranstoun. The captain, according to his sweetheart, persuaded her to give her father what was described as a love philter, saying this would make him acceptable to the old gentleman. At the captain's direction, the powder was allegedly fed to Mr. Blandy, first in tea and then in gruel. He became deathly ill, as did two maidservants who also partook. The young women noticed a white powder in the bottom of the pan of gruel, which was saved. A week later Mr. Blandy was dead.

One of the two doctors who appeared at the trial as an expert witness was Dr. Anthony Addington, a prominent physician. He had cared for Mr. Blandy in his last illness and had suspected poisoning because of the inflammation of his patient's tongue and throat, his inability to swallow, his weak, irregular pulse and respiration, and the diarrhea and perianal ulcers which developed. Addington told how one of the maids saw Miss Blandy throw a paper into the fire; the

11. Parry, 1925: p. 221; McElwee, 1952: pp. 190–91; deFord, 1960: pp. 54, 60; Davison, 1964; White, 1965: pp. 40, 78–79, 110–16, 154, 192; Campbell, 1981.

suspicious servant snatched it out and later gave the paper to the physician. Inside he found "a whiteish powder, like white arsenic in taste, but slightly discoloured by a little burnt paper mixed with it. I cannot swear this powder was arsenic, or any other poison, because the quantity was too small to make any experiment with it that could be depended on." A second physician confirmed the symptoms described by Dr. Addington.

On cross-examination, the latter testified that he believed powder found in the bottom of the pan of water gruel to be arsenic because it was white, gritty, insipid, insoluble in cold water, and released an odor of garlic when thrown on a red-hot iron. In addition, he noted, the substance reacted to a precipitation test in the same way as did a known sample of arsenic purchased from a druggist. The nonspecifity of these tests is notable.

Addington had performed an autopsy on the day after death, observing external lividity, discoloration of the lungs, liver, spleen, and kidneys, extreme inflammation of the interior of the stomach and duodenum and of the whites of the eyes, and not "the least trace of a natural decay in any part whatsoever," a reference to the supposed preservative effect of arsenic. Neither organs nor stomach contents were tested for poison. Mary Blandy admitted giving the powder to her father but stated that she did not know it was poison. She was hanged.[12] No action was taken against Captain Cranstoun, seemingly because there was only Mary Blandy's word that he had been an accomplice.

Eliza Fenning was tried in 1815 for the attempted murder of her master and mistress and of the master's father. Her apparent motivation was a severe reprimand for misbehavior by her mistress. Within a few minutes after the older members of the household and Eliza began to eat the dumplings she had made, they noticed a burning sensation in their throats. Soon they and she vomited and their eyes became inflamed.

Full of suspicion, the mistress recalled that arsenic for use as mouse poison was kept in an unlocked desk drawer in the house. She therefore saved the unwashed mixing bowl and the remainder of the dumplings. Further, she later testified, she noticed that the knives and forks used to eat the dumplings were blackened.

12. J. G. Smith, 1825: pp. 198–205; Glaister, 1897, 1960; Lee, 1909: pp. 32–33; Roughead, 1914: pp. 57–58, 80–86; Davison, 1964.

On the following day Mr. John Marshall, a surgeon who had been called in to treat the sick people,

> examined the dish; I washed it with a tea-kettle of warm water, I first stirred it, and let it subside; I decanted it off, I found half a tea spoon of white powder; I washed it a second time; I decidedly found it to be arsenic.
>
> *Q*. Will arsenic if it is cut with a knife, will it produce on the knife the colour of blackness?—*A*. I have no doubt of it: I examined the yeast; there was no arsenic in that.

Marshall added that he was sure the symptoms exhibited by his patients were caused by arsenic. On the basis of this uncertain and partly subjective evidence, Eliza Fenning was found guilty, was sentenced to death (*OB,* April 1815: pp. 220–23; Davison, 1964), and was executed.

It is refreshing to note that one John Watkins, a historian and biographer without scientific training, in a book published in the same year on the Fenning case demolished the validity of much of Marshall's testimony and castigated the surgeon for his inaccuracy and carelessness. The latter had estimated that there was a half teaspoonful of the poison in the residue of dough left in the mixing dish after the dumplings were made. Watkins calculated that if this were so, since cooks customarily leave little residue in such a dish, the entire mass of dough *before* the dumplings were formed must have contained 1,800 grams of arsenic!

> Mr. M. found it to be *arsenic,* but he has not stated how he *knew* it to be so. Did Mr. M., by mere inspection, find it to be so? Or did he find it to be so on the authority of any other person? Did he *test* it, and when? What *tests* did he use? What *became* of the arsenic? . . . Was the dish the only vessel, except the flour-tub and yeast-basin, that Mr. M. examined? Did it not occur to him to examine the pot in which the dumplings were boiled? What became of the water they were boiled in? . . . Did Mr. M. inquire, where the water was got from that the dumplings were mixed with, and did he inspect the vessel it was fetched in? Did he examine the milk-can that hung in the kitchen? and the salt-vessel from which the salt was taken for the dumplings? Did he examine the sauce?

Watkins also arranged for the baking of a yeast dumpling containing a large amount of arsenic. Then he cut the dumpling with a clean knife. The latter did *not* turn black, nor did this happen when a paste of arsenic and water was allowed to dry on the blade. He pointed out, finally, that no poison of any kind had been demonstrated in the remainder of the dumplings baked by Eliza Fenning.[13]

In 1817, two years after Watkins's book appeared, Marshall published *Remarks on Arsenic, Considered as a Poison and a Medicine; to which are added, five cases of recovery from the poisonous effects of arsenic. Together with the tests so successfully employed for detecting the white metallic oxide; in which those satisfactory methods, peculiar to Mr. Hume, were principally adopted, confirmed, and compared with others in use.*[14] This volume seems to have been an expansion of a thirty-nine-page work published in 1815 with a similar but even more lengthy title that ended with the statement, . . . *To which are annexed many corroborating facts, never before published, relative to the guilt of Eliza Fenning.* Both books were in part a defense of Marshall's testimony at the Fenning trial. The 1817 version was reviewed in two important medical journals; in one, a critic remarked that "public opinion was very much divided respecting the guilt of this misguided female." Both viewers recognized that "the importance of forensic medicine is sufficient to direct our immediate attention to any work connected with it." The reviews, although couched in the courtly language deemed appropriate when a medical journal discussed a book by a medical man, were stingingly critical of Marshall for reasons ranging from bad chemistry to bad grammar (Review, 1817a, b).

By 1835, several precipitation tests and at least one reduction test for arsenic had been developed and described in English publications, although none of the methods was entirely specific.[15] Then in 1836 James Marsh, employed as a chemist at the Royal Arsenal in Woolwich and as an assistant to Michael Faraday at the Woolwich Military Academy, described his new reduction test. With it he was able "to separate very minute quantities of arsenic from gruel, soup, porter, and other alimentary liquors"—in other words, from the stomach contents of a poisoning victim. He could, he said, detect as little as 1/120 of a grain (0.5 mgm) of an arsenic compound and reported that his test was unambiguous providing that precautions were taken so that the zinc used in the reaction was not itself contaminated with arsenic (Marsh, 1836).

13. Watkins (1815). The forensic medical specialist John G. Smith, who quoted this passage (1825: pp. 207–11), fully agreed with Watkins's conclusions.

14. Marshall (1817). The title refers to Hume's test for arsenic, a precipitation method (Campbell, 1965).

15. S. Farr, 1819: pp. 52–53; J. G. Smith, 1821: pp. 91–93; Dunglison, 1827: p. 29; Campbell, 1965; Thorwald, 1965: pp. 274–75.

The Marsh test received a good deal of publicity, not all of it favorable, in connection with the Lafarge poisoning case in France in 1840. Meanwhile the chemist had been conscientiously trying to improve his method. Then in 1841 Hugo Reinsch published a new test for arsenic. This procedure in turn was criticized in connection with the Smethurst poisoning trial in 1859 (see below). Doubts that arose about both tests appear to have been due not to inadequacies of method but to contaminated reagents.[16] In any case, both procedures soon appeared in textbooks of forensic medicine.[17]

Application of the Marsh test was reported in testimony at the Old Bailey as early as 1839. A chemist used the test on stomach contents but failed to detect arsenic. However, since he stated that the method "is supposed to detect the 500,000th part of a grain," one wonders whether he really understood the procedure (*CB,* Aug. 1839: pp. 631–39). Use of both the Marsh and Reinsch methods was described again in court in 1846 (*OB,* Aug. 1839: pp. 631–39; May 1846: pp. 143–59), but testimony by experts at four subsequent trials for murder by arsenic omitted specific mention of either procedure (*OB,* Sept. 1847: pp. 1023–37; Dec. 1847: pp. 338–58; Aug. 1848: pp. 562–73; June 1849: pp. 148–55).

Ann Merritt was tried in 1850 for murdering her husband by feeding him gruel containing arsenic. She had prepared the food herself, and he had eaten it about a quarter past eleven in the morning. Soon afterward he grew sick, and died just after midnight of the same day.

The husband, it seems, was very fond of a drink made from effervescing soda and acid powders. Mrs. Merritt claimed that she had placed the unlabeled paper of poison in a cupboard among her husband's powders. In the unlikely case that the jurymen could be convinced that she had acted innocently and that the husband had by accident taken noneffervescing arsenic instead of soda and acid, the wife might have been found guilty on the lesser charge of manslaughter. Thus a crucial forensic medical question arose: Was the time interval between the husband's ingestion of the poison and his death so long that he could have taken the arsenic himself during the night, roughly twenty-four hours before his death, or was the poison in his wife's gruel which he ate late the next morning, about thirteen hours before his death?

16. S. Smith, 1928; Gettler, 1956; Campbell, 1965, 1981; Thorwald, 1965: pp. 274–92.

17. Taylor, 1844b: p. 538; 1848: pp. 281–88; Christison, 1845: pp. 206, 212–18.

Dr. Henry Letheby testified that he had analyzed a portion of the liver and estimated that the entire organ contained about two grains of arsenic. The stomach, he said, held eight and a half grains, but there was little poison in the intestines. He concluded from this that the arsenic had been swallowed two or three hours before death. Ann Merritt was condemned to the gallows (*OB,* Mar. 1850: pp. 524–34).

However, a "medical man of large experience"[18] was astounded at Letheby's estimate of when the poison had been ingested, as were other authorities. Their reasons were that two grains of arsenic, a lethal amount, could not have accumulated in the liver in such a short time, that digestion of food by a stomach inflamed by arsenic could take eight hours or more, that purging might have cleared the intestines of poison, and that the stomach contents observed at autopsy had been described as "slightly pink," a color not characteristic of gruel but perhaps due to gastric bleeding resulting from prolonged inflammation. These objections were communicated to the sheriffs, and ultimately the evidence in the case was referred to Sir Benjamin Brodie, Dr. Billing, Dr. Leeson, and other prominent medical men. They could not agree on the time when the poison must have been ingested. Under some urging, Letheby finally wrote to the Home Secretary, conceding that it was possible or even probable "that the arsenic might have been taken, as the woman asserted, early in the morning of her husband's death." The upshot was that the capital sentence was commuted to one of penal servitude for life.

The need for reliable tests for poison and for understanding and skill in their employment was emphasized again at the trial of Thomas Smethurst. The details of the notorious "Richmond case," as it was sometimes known, have been recounted several times and will only be summarized here.[19] In August 1859 Smethurst was put on trial for the murder by poison of Isabella Bankes, a lady of some means, whom he had bigamously married the preceding December. The indictment for murder grew out of testimony at the inquest by Dr. Alfred Swaine Taylor that his tests had shown arsenic in the woman's body, and indeed under the microscope he had seen crystals of the poison on the copper gauze that was employed in the Reinsch tests. However, at the trial Taylor admitted that he had been at fault and that the arsenic had not come from the body but rather was a contaminant of the gauze.

18. Browne and Stewart (1883: pp. 364–72), who relate the events subsequent to the trial, do not identify this individual.

19. *OB,* Aug. 1859: pp. 504–87; Browne and Stewart, 1883: pp. 448–79; Stephen, 1883: 3, 438–65; Parry, 1931; Browne and Tullett, 1951: p. 23; Glaister, 1954; Nagle, 1970.

He had used the latter in his tests, he said, for the past fourteen years, an admission about which, it has been remarked, Taylor was, perhaps fortunately, not further questioned. He also found antimony in the body of Isabella Bankes; it turned out that this substance, which is poisonous in sufficient quantity, had been an ingredient of medicines administered to her in her last illness. Autopsy findings included a uterus containing a five- to seven-week fetus. There was congestion of the stomach, inflammation of the ileum, and inflammation and ulceration of parts of the large intestine; the changes in the digestive tract were considered to have "resulted from some irritant, administered frequently during life."

Taylor's evidence and that of other expert medical witnesses, much of it contradictory, nevertheless resulted in Smethurst's conviction, and he was sentenced to the gallows. But petitions for a reprieve were presented to Lord Chief Justice Baron Pollock, the presiding judge, who recommended to the Home Secretary that the controversy be submitted to Sir Benjamin Brodie, the surgeon. He, it will be remembered, had himself many years before conducted experiments on the actions of poisons. The immediate result of this move was, as Stephen points out, that "the responsibility of the decision was thus shifted from those on whom it properly rested on to a man who, however skilled and learned as a surgeon, was neither a juryman nor a judge" (3, 464–65). Brodie, after due deliberation, found six reasons for thinking that Smethurst was guilty and eight that perhaps he was not. The surgeon concluded that "there is not absolute and complete evidence of Smethurst's guilt." Eventually he was pardoned.

Advances in medical knowledge in the century and more since this trial have made possible new theories for the cause of Miss Bankes's demise, namely that the pathological changes observed in her intestines were due not to an irritant poison but to ulcerative colitis (Davison, 1964) or to Crohn's disease (Nagle, 1970).

Not surprisingly, the Smethurst trial, like some that had preceded it, served to throw the whole subject of forensic medical testimony into doubt and disrepute. Legal and medical criticisms appeared repeatedly in the press, and years passed before public confidence in the expert medical witness was restored.

MERCURY

Old Bailey trials for murder or attempted murder by poisoning with mercury salts involved either corrosive sublimate (bichloride of mercury) or ammoniated mercury. The former is very poisonous. The latter, being poorly absorbed by the alimentary tract, is less likely to prove lethal. A third mercury compound, calomel or mercurous chloride, had widespread medicinal use as a purgative and antisyphilitic.

Charles Angus, once employed by a chemist, was accused in 1808 of the murder of Margaret Burns, half sister of Angus's deceased wife. Miss Burns, who lived with Angus as his housekeeper, had been observed by neighbors to be pregnant. She became sick on the morning of 23 March, vomiting and complaining of dysuria and acute thirst. Angus insisted on caring for her himself and did not allow his two servants to send for medical assistance. At about 10 A.M. on Friday, 25 March, she expired.

On Sunday, word of the death reached the coroner. After an autopsy it was concluded that the woman had been poisoned and also that recently she had delivered a baby. The body of the latter could not be found. An inquest led to the indictment of Angus for murder.

At his trial it was shown that he possessed a trocar, an instrument that might have been used to induce an abortion, and also a large collection of bottles. One of them contained oil of savin, sometimes used as an abortifacient; in sufficient quantity it is lethal. A physician and chemist tested the liquid in another bottle and said that they found corrosive sublimate; the method of analysis was not described. No poison was detected in the gastric contents.

In the wall of the woman's stomach was a perforation. Expert witnesses disagreed as to whether the gastric perforation and inflammation were due to poison, to disease, or to post-mortem "digestion" by gastric juices. The classic observations of Morgagni (1769) and John Hunter (1837) on this subject were invoked. Counsel for the defense sought to prove that the changes in the stomach wall had occurred only after death. The medical witness appearing for the defense claimed that the uterus did *not* show signs of recent pregnancy.

The repeated disagreements between experts testifying for the prosecution and those for the defense, together with what was virtually a directed verdict from the judge, resulted in a jury decision that Angus was not guilty. But this did not end matters, as medical witnesses for both sides soon afterward published lengthy statements in support of their testimony. There seems little doubt that Miss Burns had been pregnant and at or near term. Never really resolved, however, were questions as to whether she was given bichloride of mercury; whether, if so, it caused death; what caused the gastric pathology—and what happened to the body of the newborn baby (Forbes, 1981b).

LEAD

A young woman was poisoned with a substance dissolved in what appeared to be brandy bitters. Circumstantial evidence later suggested lead acetate, "sugar of lead." At autopsy the gastric lining exhibited inflammation and dark-colored spots. The kidneys were congested. Dr. Henry B. Leeson made an analysis, adding hydrogen sulphide to an aqueous extract of the stomach. This, he said, "yielded a black precipitate; I ultimately obtained a globule of metallic lead from the stomach." This was the test later recommended by Christison (1845: p. 398). The metallic lead Leeson recovered weighed 1.1 grain (66 mgm); he stated that this amount of lead as lead carbonate would not constitute a fatal dose. He was probably mistaken regarding the identity of the lead compound, as a paper marked "Sugar of lead-poison" was discovered in the prisoner's cupboard. He was found not guilty (*OB*, Nov. 1844: pp. 38–50).

TARTARIC ACID AND TARTAR EMETIC

Both tartaric acid and tartar emetic were involved in cases of accidental poisoning, once due to a chemist's error and once when gin purchased at a public house was put in a borrowed bottle. The tartar emetic[20] was identified by chemical analysis (*OB*, Jan. 1845: pp. 389–90; Aug. 1856: pp. 685–89).

MORISON'S PILLS

Morison's pills were the product of James Morison, a notorious and very successful London quack.[21] One of his salesmen, a "Hygeian agent" named Robert Salmon, was brought to trial in 1836 for the

20. Tartar emetic actually consists of antimony tartrate and potassium tartrate.

21. Morison, formerly a West Indian and Baltic merchant, later became a self-styled "Hygeist" who claimed that after thirty-five years of great suffering and the failure of repeated medical treatments, he had been cured by the blood- and body-purifying powers of his proprietary preparations. His "vegetable universal medicines," allegedly remedies for fevers, smallpox, measles, consumption, debility, and all other ills, were manufactured at an establishment at 33 Euston Road, London, which he called the British College of Health. The single tax stamp required on each box of medicine cost Morison 1 ½ *d.*; such was his commercial success that he paid £60,000 to the British government just for stamps between 1830 and 1840 (James Morison, 1840; Peterson, 1973; Helfand, 1974).

manslaughter death of Captain John Mackenzie, aged thirty-two, master of a merchant ship. The captain, after initial skepticism, had been buying Morison's pills from Salmon and another agent, first as "an opening medicine" (laxative) and later for rheumatism in his knee. The pills were sold as No. 1 and No. 2; these were not to be taken separately. Mackenzie's knee became more painful; instead of abandoning the medication he increased the dose on Salmon's direction, soon taking fifteen to twenty pills daily. The patient's condition grew steadily worse, and he was unable to retain food because of constant bloody vomiting and purging. A surgeon-apothecary and a consulting physician were called in but did not succeed in persuading the dying Mackenzie to stop taking Morison's pills. A day or two later the captain had succumbed.

Post-mortem dissection revealed marked inflammation and ulceration of the stomach and intestines, almost to the point of gangrene. The medical men at the autopsy were sure that these changes were recent and not of long standing. All other organs were healthy. The right knee showed changes characteristic of rheumatism.

An incomplete analysis of the pills indicated the presence of cream of tartar (potassium bitartrate), aloes, gamboge (a yellow resin used by artists as a pigment and by apothecaries as a very powerful cathartic), and a little asafoetida.[22] According to the testimony of the analytical chemist, the proportions of the ingredients were different in the No. 1 and No. 2 pills, as were the sizes of the pills, which apparently weighed between three and four grains each. Cream of tartar is a mild laxative. Aloes is very strong. The fatal dose of gamboge may be as little as 1 gram (15.4 grains), and the substance is now regarded as too hazardous for use as a medicine (Dreisbach, 1980: pp. 429–30).

Salmon's defense, occupying more than six closely printed pages of the *Sessions Papers,* was a triumph of obfuscation, self-justification, and pretended virtue:

> The doctors of the present day designate Harvey, the great discoverer of the circulation of the blood, immortal; but they know that their medical forefathers considered him a quack, and persecuted him, because he had been bold enough to declare a great truth, which truth was opposed to their preconceived notions—the public are now beginning to see that they are the greatest quacks who cannot cure their

22. Morison, of course, tried to keep his formulas a secret. Some pharmacopoeias state that the pills contained in addition jalap resin, colocynth, rhubarb, and myrrh. Available recipes disagree with regard to both ingredients and amounts. Individual pills are known to have varied considerably in weight (Helfand, 1974).

> patients; and they the best physicians who can cure them, whether licensed or unlicensed.

But the most remarkable testimony was yet to come. A procession of no less than twenty-five character witnesses entered the witness box, one by one, to relate how Morison's pills had cured them and their children of brief or lengthy ills ranging from stricture, ulcerated sore throat, gallstones, and hemorrhoids to fistula, smallpox, and rupture. Satisfied consumers included tradesmen, a clergyman, and a surgeon of long experience. This last gentleman had at various times, he said, been cured of rheumatic gout, liver disease, erysipelas, and epilepsy, all by dint of taking up to seventy-five Morison's pills a day. A cheesemonger stated that in two years he had consumed twenty thousand at a cost of £22. A "practising Hygeist," a former teacher of English grammar, related that during a cholera epidemic at Carlisle he had cured between one hundred fifty and two hundred victims with Morison's pills, which he was then selling.

Testimony disclosed that the defendant, Salmon, sold the pills but "took no money for his attendance." Thus, although the quack did not hesitate to prescribe for any illness, a simple matter since his prescription was always basically the same, he never exposed himself to the charge of practicing medicine *for a fee;* "he gave his advice quite gratuitously" (*OB,* April 1836: pp. 904–36).

It all helped. Salmon was let off with a fine of £200.

This was not the first time a "Hygeist" had been in trouble with the law. Another saleman was tried in 1834 in York for the death by manslaughter of a young man who had purchased and consumed daily doses of ten, fifteen, and twenty Morison's pills as a treatment for smallpox. Autopsy findings included inflammation of the stomach and intestines. The accused quack was found guilty and sentenced to six months in prison (Morison's, 1834). In 1836 the deaths of at least three victims of the pills in addition to Captain Mackenzie were reported (Death, 1836; Morison's 1836a,b,c; Allnatt).

SAVIN

Savin is an oil from *Juniperus sabina.* A married man was tried for administering the substance in pills to a young woman, not his wife, to procure an abortion. She became ill. A surgeon who examined her could not, on the basis of the girl's description, identify the active agent in the pill but stated that he found her weak and debilitated, a condition which "might follow from the taking of two pills containing a powerful irritant poison." In spite of this uncertain evidence the accused was sent to prison for six years, a penalty reflecting the court's strong disapproval of this offense (*OB,* April 1855: pp. 678–82).

LOBELIA

Lobelia, an American plant, was used in medicine as an emetic, expectorant, and cathartic. Fatalities following its administration resulted in two trials for manslaughter. Lobelia was an ingredient of a "composition powder" administered in solution as an enema to a thirteen-year-old boy. Post-mortem examination showed that the left side of the chest was filled with fluid, the left lung was compressed, and the stomach and intestines, particularly the rectum, were grealy inflamed. The pathologic changes in the chest were not considered to be a result of the enema. When Henry Letheby examined a sample of the composition powder, he definitely identified ginger and cayenne pepper. There was, he said, "no positive test for lobelia; but as far as the microscope would guide me, I believe it to have been lobelia," an interesting early reference to forensic use of this instrument. In tests on himself, he found that the powder was very irritating to the inside of his mouth and even to the back of his hand. Letheby regarded lobelia as a dangerous drug (*OB,* Aug. 1851: pp. 526–32).

In a second manslaughter trial the physician-chemist ascribed severe gastric inflammation and ulceration in a woman to the ingestion of a mixture containing cayenne pepper and, by his analysis, 110 grains of lobelia seed (*OB,* Feb. 1853: pp. 475–80).

STRYCHNINE

Strychnine, commonly a component of rat and mouse poison, was administered medically in paralytic affections, chronic diarrhea, and dysentery. Strychnine is the principal alkaloid in *nux vomica* seeds, also used medicinally. Although the seeds had long been known, strychnine as such was not discovered until 1818, appearing relatively late on the toxicological scene. The substance is crystalline, almost insoluble in water, bitter, and extremely poisonous. Strychnine markedly increases the reflex excitability of the medulla oblongata and spinal cord; as a result, convulsions and generalized tetanic seizures occur. The victim is unable to breathe and death results (Dreisbach, 1980: pp. 411–12). Because of its insolubility, as Robinson (1856) pointed out, it was not always possible to be sure how much of the strychnine ingested in a mixture had been absorbed in the digestive tract. He urged the medical practitioner investigating a fatal case of suspected strychnine poisoning to test for the substance in any residue of food or drink, in appropriate body organs, and in the vomitus and excreta. Taylor described microscopic and chemical tests for strychnine which he regarded as specific (1848: pp. 622–24).

One of Britain's most notorious murder trials took place at the Old Bailey in May 1856.[23] The victim was John Parsons Cook. The defendant was William Palmer, a thirty-one-year-old married surgeon of Rugeley. After a good beginning in his profession, he had come to spend more and more time at the racetrack and finally gave up his practice. By 1854, deeply in debt, he insured his wife's life for £13,000. Nine months later she died. The insurance company paid the full amount, but in the following months Palmer was unable to obtain a life insurance policy for £80,000 on his brother, a hopeless alcoholic. An attempt to insure the life of a farm employee was also unsuccessful. By November 1855 Palmer's debts amounted to £12,500. In the last two years he had in addition repeatedly forged his mother's name on bills and Cook's name on checks.

The latter individual, genial, well-to-do, healthy, and a little younger than his close friend Palmer, was also becoming a racing enthusiast. On 13 November 1855 Cook won £2,050 at the track. Palmer, now almost penniless, had a motive for murder. His medical knowledge suggested a means, and the fact that the two men shared rooms, first near the racetrack in Shrewsbury and subsequently in Rugeley, provided the opportunity.

Events hereafter became complicated. In summary, evidence at the trial showed that Palmer, seldom far from Cook, repeatedly found pretexts when they were alone to give him drinks of brandy, coffee, or broth. Shortly afterward Cook would complain of a bitter, burning sensation in his throat, and would often vomit. Palmer, acting as Cook's physician, ascribed this to illness, then persuaded his patient to drink further liquids as restoratives. A servant girl who sampled some of the broth sent by Palmer to his friend was also made sick. There was

23. *OB,* May 1856: pp. 5–224; Browne and Stewart, 1883: pp. 85–232; Stephen, 1883: pp. 389–425; Waldo, 1904: pp. 176–82; Knott and Watson, 1923; Glaister, 1956; Davison, 1964.

evidence that Palmer was giving the young man tartar emetic in amounts to make him ill; the effect was both to simulate a disease and to weaken Cook. Indeed, he was examined several times by an eighty-year-old local practitioner, who found the patient free of fever and with a good pulse. This doctor suggested that the persistent vomiting was due to overindulgence in wine.

Palmer found time to go to London where, stating that he was acting on behalf of Cook, he obtained some of the latter's funds which Palmer used to satisfy certain of his debtors. He then returned to Rugeley. The aged local doctor again prescribed pills to the sick man. At midnight the victim, experiencing violent spasms, awakened the household with his screams.

For the next several days, the patient alternated between bouts of severe illness, each of them following the administration of drink or medicine by Palmer, and periods of partial recovery. During his attacks he repeatedly called out for assistance. On Tuesday, 20 November, Palmer went to the shop of the Rugeley chemist and purchased prussic acid, strychnine, and liquor of opium in the form of Batley's sedative. About 10:30 P.M. he administered more pills, again supposedly furnished by the local doctor. At approximately midnight Cook, after another violent tetanic seizure, died quietly. A few days later the same local physician issued a death certificate, listing apoplexy as the cause.

At the post-mortem examination, which was conducted on 26 November by two physicians and a surgeon, Palmer was present. Dr. Harland, one of those who performed the autopsy, later testified that, in effect, the body did not show signs of disease that would account for death. The appearance of the stomach and intestines was not remarkable. Spleen, pancreas, lungs, and heart seemed healthy. The right kidney was enlarged and soft. Two months after death the body was exhumed and another autopsy was performed. At that time it was noted that the brain and spinal cord and their investments also seemed healthy.

While the stomach and intestines were being removed at the first post-mortem examination, Palmer managed to jostle one of the participants so that some stomach contents were spilled into the abdomen. The organs were then placed in a jar covered with two layers of bladder that were tightly tied in place. Later it was discovered that the container was missing. When it was found outside the room, the protective cover had been slashed in two places. A new cover was applied, and the whole was sent to Alfred Swaine Taylor for examination, although not before Palmer had attempted unsuccessfully to bribe a postboy to upset the fly in which the jar was to be started on its journey to London.

There an inquest was called. Palmer promptly wrote to the coroner and sent him gifts of game. The poisoner also managed to persuade the local postmaster to open a letter from Taylor to Cook's father-in-law and disclose its contents. Thus Palmer learned of Taylor's report that, except for a trace of antimony, no strychnine or other poison had been discovered in the organs. Nonetheless, when the inquest was held on 26 November, the coroner's jury rendered a verdict of wilful murder against Palmer.

At the trial Taylor disclosed the condition of the viscera when the jar was opened:

> The stomach had been completely cut from end to end; all the contents were gone, and the fine mucous surface, on which any poison if present would be found, was lying in contact with the outsides of the intestines, all thrown together. . . . In journeying up to London it must have been shaken in every possible way. At my request other portions of the body were sent—the liver, the spleen, and the two kidneys; in addition, a small bottle of blood, unlabelled, giving us no idea whence it was taken.

Palmer's trial was characterized by contradictory forensic medical testimony. Twenty-four medicolegal experts appeared for the prosecution, among them such figures as Thomas Blizzard Curling,[24] Sir Benjamin Brodie, Alfred Swaine Taylor, and Sir Robert Christison. Fifteen expert witnesses, including Henry Letheby, testified for the defense. In the view of Professor John Glaister (1956), a twentieth-century British forensic medical specialist, three principal medicolegal questions were at issue. The prosecution asserted that Cook had been poisoned with strychnine; why was this not detected by expert and sensitive analysis in his body? About one hour intervened between Palmer's alleged administration of strychnine pills to Cook and the onset of symptoms that ended in his death; was such a delay characteristic of the action of this poison? Finally, was death due to poison or to disease?

Evidence from experiments with rabbits poisoned with strychnine was cited to show that the poison could not always be detected in their bodies. A similar finding in known cases of human strychnine poison-

24. Curling (1811–88), still a young man, was later to make a reputation for describing the acute duodenal ulcer that may follow severe burns and for suggesting that cretinism may be due to thyroid deficiency.

ing was mentioned. (It is now recognized that the poison is rapidly metabolized, about three-fourths of it disappearing from the blood stream, but not necessarily from the organs, in one hundred minutes.) As Glaister (1956) points out, the failure to detect strychnine in Cook's body seemed to support both the prosecution's contention that this was to be expected and the defense's argument that the poison had never been administered.

The Crown insisted, and witnesses for Palmer's defense denied, that the time of onset of symptoms before death was consistent with the time at which, it was alleged, Palmer had given pills to Cook on the evening of 20 November.

The third issue, whether death was the result of poison or disease, provoked lengthy disputation. Taylor, Sir Benjamin Brodie, and other witnesses for the prosecution denied the allegation that the circumstances and symptoms preceding Cook's death could have been due to tetanus or epilepsy. In tetanus, it was emphasized, lockjaw appears early and regularly, remissions are brief, and the disease is usually terminated in twenty-four to forty-eight hours. Epileptic convulsions are never tetanic, and the epileptic patient loses consciousness during a seizure. Sir Benjamin Brodie emphasized that Cook's symptoms did not conform to those of any disease in his experience, and three expert witnesses for the defense agreed.

Neither side denied that antimony had at first been given to Cook, that it would account for all the earlier symptoms of his illness—for example, before the appearance of the convulsions—and that Palmer had given the antimony as cream of tartar.

Lord Chief Justice Campbell delivered a lengthy charge to the jury, reminding its members that they must regard the accused as if he were innocent and should concentrate their attention on the evidence as to the crime itself:

> The great question that I propounded for your consideration was whether Cook's symptoms were consistent with strychnia, and if they were not, then the conclusion would be in favour of the prisoner; but if they were consistent with strychnia, then you are not upon that alone to find a verdict of guilty against him; but you are to consider the other evidence and see whether the death arose from strychnia or not. . . .
>
> Gentlemen, the case is now in your hands; and, unless upon the part of the prosecution a clear conviction has been brought to your minds of the guilt of the prisoner, it is your duty to acquit him. You are not to proceed even upon a strong suspicion; there must be the strongest conviction in your minds that he was guilty of this offense;

> and if there be any reasonable doubt remaining in your mind, you will give him the benefit of that doubt; but if you come to a clear conviction that he was guilty, you will not be deterred from doing your duty by any considerations as have been suggested to you.

After deliberating for an hour and eighteen minutes, the jury returned a verdict of guilty. Palmer was executed on 14 June 1856.

The Palmer poisoning case is famous in the history of British crime. Much less well known are some important details relating to the deaths of the murderer's wife and brother. Ann Palmer had died on 29 September 1854, and Walter Palmer on 16 August 1855. The inquest into Cook's death was held on 26 November 1855. Evidently the decision of the coroner's jury to indict William Palmer for the wilful murder of Cook prompted the police to wonder what had caused the two rather recent sudden deaths within the family. The bodies of Ann and Walter were exhumed about three weeks after the inquest on Cook, and careful post-mortem examinations were conducted by Dr. David H. Monckton on 21 and 22 December. His meticulous autopsy report and his testimony at the subsequent inquest were published in the *Lancet* (Monckton, 1856). In effect, he found no real evidence that Walter Palmer had been poisoned. Monckton listed a number of organs that he had removed and sent to Alfred Swaine Taylor for examination.[25]

Monckton's post-mortem examination of the exhumed body of Ann Palmer was also careful (Monckton, 1856). He set aside portions of several organs for analysis and study by Taylor. At the coroner's inquest into Mrs. Palmer's death, Monckton testified that he found no evidence as to the cause of death; the digestive tract appeared to be healthy. Taylor's toxicological analysis of Mrs. Palmer's organs, however, yielded some positive results (Taylor and Rees, 1856). He testified, "On the stomach at its greater end, and on the outside, there was a yellowish-coloured streak, which, when examined with a magnifying glass, presented the appearance of mineral matter. It was such an appearance as I have never seen in twenty-five year's experience, except when mineral poison was in the stomach."

Taylor examined stomach, small and large intestines, kidneys, liver, heart, lungs, and spleen. Antimony and a minute amount of arsenic were detected in the viscera examined and in the blood. On the basis of relative amounts of the poison in various anatomical locations, Taylor and his assistant expressed the opinion that the antimony

25. A report of Taylor's findings could not be located.

had been taken in doses at intervals for several days. They could not be certain that it had caused death.

Pressed in cross-examination as to whether there was a lethal amount of antimony in the body, Taylor made an important toxicological observation: "The effects of poison upon the system do not depend upon the quantity taken into the stomach, but upon the quantity absorbed into the system. It is not five or fifty grains in the stomach that are decisive, but the quantity which impregnates the blood. . . . That which we find in the stomach is only the sediment or dregs of what has killed." It was his final conclusion that Ann Palmer "died from the effects of tartar emetic, and no other cause, after antimony." Stephen states that a true bill, that is, a bill of indictment endorsed by the grand jury when it is satisfied of the truth of an accusation, was returned against William Palmer. But he had already been convicted of Cook's death, and no further steps were taken (1883, p. 389).

Taylor's testimony illustrates both the advances that he and a few others had achieved in forensic toxicology and pathology and the important contributions that could be made by a properly qualified and motivated expert. Had more of his contemporaries taken advantage of his teachings, the progress of English forensic medicine would have been much more rapid.

COCCULUS INDICUS

Cocculus indicus is a name for dried berries from the East Indian climbing vine *Anamirta cocculus*. The highly poisonous fruit has been dropped in streams to stupefy fish and added as an illegal adulterant to porter and beer, either to increase their intoxicating effect or, according to Christison, to substitute for hops, since the berries contributed a bitter taste. Apparently the amount absorbed by drugged fish was not sufficient to render their flesh poisonous (Christison, 1845: pp. 696–98). An active principle in the berry is picrotoxin, or cocculin, a powerful poison with an action similar to that of strychnine.

One September morning in 1846 it was discovered that a poacher had been busy in the waters of Her Majesty's river, the Hampton Court Cut, and that dozens of fish lay dead or dying. Henry Jepson, a Hampton surgeon, told later in court how he collected several of the fish and, in a rather unusual medicolegal investigation, "found the stomachs of three of them stained with a deep yellow matter, which is a peculiar property of the cocculus indicus; two others were gorged with a paste" made from the berries. A youth convicted of the poisoning was sentenced to transportation for seven years (*OB*, Sept. 1846: pp. 747–48).

OPIUM AND ITS DERIVATIVES

Opium, an ancient and widely used narcotic and analgesic, is a gum or resin made by air-drying the juice of poppy capsules, *Papaver somniferum*. Morphia or morphine is a white alkaloid extracted from opium. Because of its insolubility in water, morphine is often prepared as a soluble salt, for example, morphine sulfate. By modern definition laudanum is a tincture of opium, but in the seventeenth century "laudanum" also designated a pill mass containing opium. Thomas Sydenham (1624–89) mentioned such a medication as well as syrup of poppies and paregoric, an opium-containing soothing syrup (Kramer, 1979).

Opium preparations were widely employed in medicine in the seventeenth, eighteenth, and nineteenth centuries despite the recognition that their habitual use could lead to addiction. According to Lomax, in the nineteenth century opiates "were as readily available as aspirin today, and just as cheap" (1973). At midcentury Taylor stated that laudanum was sold at retail to the public at rates of "from half a drachm [1.85 cc.] to two drachms for twopence, from two drachms to four drachms for fourpence,—exceeding this quantity, eightpence and one shilling per ounce."[26] Opiates were swallowed to relieve pain, worry, or boredom, to ward off fevers, to treat sickness, to induce euphoria, and to satisfy addiction. Measures even for partial control of the sale of opium and its derivatives were not introduced until 1868, when the Pharmacy Act was passed.[27] It is not surprising that, as we have observed (table 6), overdoses of this drug were a leading cause of poison deaths in England and Wales in 1837–38.

Soothing mixtures with an opiate base that were commonly and freely administered to babies and children included "Godfrey's Cordial" (composed of sassafras, treacle, and tincture of opium), "Mrs. Winslow's Soothing Syrup," also known as "Quietness" (nearly one

26. A typical urban semi-skilled worker in 1841 paid 8-1/2*d*. for a loaf of bread, 5*d*. for a pound of meat, and 9*d*. for a pound of butter (Burnett, 1969: p. 263).

27. Lomax, 1973; Berridge, 1979; Peters, 1981.

grain of morphine per ounce of syrup),[28] "Dalby's Carminative" (oils of peppermint, nutmeg, and aniseed, aromatic tinctures, magnesium carbonate, and tincture of opium), "Black Drop" (opium and morphia in wild crab juice), "Locock's Pulmonic Wafers," "Dover's Powder" (opium, ipecac, and, originally, liquorice),[29] "Battley's Sedative Liquor" (solution of opium in vegetable acids), "Chlorodyne" (chloroform, oil of peppermint, hydrocyanic acid, and morphine hydrochloride), elixir of paregoric (alcohol, opium, benzoic acid, oil of aniseed, and camphor), and opium cough lozenges.[30] Apparently, the taste of most of these preparations was not unpleasant and they were readily acceptable to children.

As a result, accidental and—as we have seen—deliberate overdosing, particularly of small children, became all too common. Patent medicines containing opiates kept infants quiet when they were ill, troublesome, or left alone for several hours by working or drinking parents. Soothing syrups minimized the labors of baby farmers and provided a nearly undetectable method for ending infant lives. Who was to know, or knowing, to prove what had happened?[31]

A trial for murder by poisoning with laudanum occurred in Glasgow as early as 1800. An autopsy of the victim had not been performed until two weeks after death,

> at which time no appearances of poison were seen; no experiment, however, was made, in order to ascertain whether laudanum had been given to the deceased, as by that time the physicians were of opinion no laudanum, had it been administered, could have been discovered in the stomach;—the deceased had been ailing before, though not dangerously ill;—no medical person had been called during her last illness, and there was no evidence as to the manner of her death. On the other hand, it was clearly proved that the prisoner had bought great quantities of laudanum, and, as it appeared, under false pretenses. . . .

28. In 1808 it was estimated that "upwards of 200 lbs. of opium, and above 600 pints of Godfrey's cordial, are retailed to the poorer classes in the year in Nottingham" (Clarke, 1808). A druggist in Manchester did not deny that his weekly sales of Godfrey's Cordial amounted to a half a gallon and of Quietness to five or six gallons. Mrs. Winslow's Soothing Syrup originated in the United States (Havard, 1960: pp. 53–54; Lomax, 1973). The record of abuse of sedatives for children and adults is appalling (F. B. Smith, 1979: pp. 95–99).

29. Thomas Dover (1660–1742) as a youth lived for a time in the house of the renowned Dr. Thomas Sydenham. Later Dover served as physician and surgeon on a privateer.

30. Christison, 1845: p. 531; Taylor, 1848: pp. 489–91; Woodman and Tidy, 1877: pp. 331–32.

31. Havard, 1960: pp. 53–54; Langer, 1974; Lomax, 1974; Kramer, 1979.

On the want, however, of any evidence as the *corpus delicti,* the Court directed the Jury to acquit. (Burnett, 1811: p. 549)

Trials at the Old Bailey for poisoning by opium and its derivatives seem not to have occurred until the nineteenth century. Medical men had long prescribed opiates for therapeutic purposes; it may be that the direct sale of opiates to laymen without a prescription did not become common until the 1800s. Or perhaps official awareness of the lethal potential of the drug was not awakened until then. In any case, although the Old Bailey saw no trial for the felonious administration of opiates until 1838, between then and 1877 there were ten such trials. These amounted to 16 percent of all the London poisoning cases during this period.

The prisoner in the 1838 case was accused of having administered laudanum to his common-law wife. According to him, he and the victim had been living together in total poverty, finally pawning even their bedclothes. With their last coins he purchased a total of about 160 drops, or roughly 6 cc., of laudanum in two chemists' and one surgeon's shop. The couple, he related in court, consumed all the liquid, intending to commit suicide. After some hours he awoke to find the woman dead and left hurriedly. In the morning her body was discovered, as were two vials, one marked "Poison" and the other "Laudanum, poison." The containers were traced to the shops where they had been procured. Two surgeons performed an autopsy the same morning. They "examined the stomach and intestines with care—I could find no traces of laudanum—I found nothing but the remains of the ordinary food she had taken—I found nothing of a deleterious character, nor anything to induce me to suppose she had taken poison. . . . there was no smell of laudanum in the contents of the stomach." The surgeons decided that apoplexy, perhaps the result of the ingestion of laudanum, had caused death. The mother of the accused stated that her son was mentally deranged.

Here is a case in which the only test for the drug was the sense of smell. The jury must have been swayed by the circumstantial evidence; the prisoner, aged twenty-one, was found guilty and was hanged (*OB,* April 1838: pp. 1048–55).

A decade later an expert told in court how he had tested for opium:

I am a lecturer on practical chemistry at St. Thomas's Hospital. I received from Pollard a cup and basin, and analysed the contents—I found in the cup a small portion of a dark-coloured substance, which appeared to have been coarsely powdered. . . . it smelt strongly of

> opium, and had every character of crude powdered opium—I submitted it to a very careful analysis, and from it produced morphia, which is the active principle of opium; and also meconic acid, which is a substance which has never yet been found in anything but opium. . . . I found about half a grain of crude opium in the cup. (*OB*, Jan. 1848: pp. 458–62)

In a later laudanum poisoning case Henry Letheby made a remark of significance for forensic toxicologists of his time:

> Q. Assuming that the death was caused by laudanum, are you, from the quantity you find in the stomach, able to form an opinion as to the quantity that was administered? *A*. No; the action of a poison is upon the brain, and it must reach the brain before it produces its effect, and when it gets into the brain we can no longer find it; that, therefore, which is in the stomach is not that which has killed. (*OB*, July 1861: pp. 280–84)

DIGITALIS

Foxglove, *Digitalis purpurea,* contains the important drug digitalis, a powerful cardiac stimulant. It was popularized as a diuretic by William Withering.[32]

In October 1826 Jacob Evans, a quack and the author of a book on herbs, undertook the treatment of a seventeen-year-old apprentice to a cabinet maker. The youth had suffered for several weeks from severe bouts of giddiness. Evans boiled two or threepenny worth of foxglove in a quart of water until the volume was reduced to little over half a pint. "And then, my boy, you will take half of that quantity; it will make you very sick, and work you upwards and downwards." Within half an hour the patient was violently ill.

The next morning a surgeon was called; he observed symptoms of a massive dose of foxglove—a slow, weak, irregular pulse, cold extremities, coma, and absence of a pupillary reflex—"I had the room darkened, called for a candle, and found the pupil would not contract and dilate." The youth died two or three hours later. An autopsy disclosed no signs of disease. The surgeon calculated that the patient had drunk about five and a half ounces of the decoction; a few drops, he said, would have been a proper dose. The prisoner was found not

32. A physician, botanist, and mineralogist, Withering (1741–99) first learned of the value of the herb in dropsy; later he tried the remedy in the treatment of heart disease. His *Account of the Foxglove and Some of Its Medical Uses* (1785) is a classic.

guilty of a charge of murder (*OB,* Oct. 1826: pp. 777–78). Taylor, commenting on the case, says that the accused was acquitted "because he had only given his advice on the application of friends of the deceased!" (1856: p. 165).

BELLADONNA

Deadly nightshade, *Atropa belladonna,* contains hyoscyamine, which may be converted to an isomer, atropine, an important drug and, like the belladonna plant, in sufficient amount a lethal substance.

Thomas Parker was fatally poisoned by ingesting shiny black belladonna berries, sold to his wife by James Hillard, a peddler who said they were nettle berries or whortleberries.[33] Tarts made from the berries poisoned husband and wife. Next morning both were taken unconscious to the London Hospital. An apothecary who attended the husband before his death testified that the "symptoms were as if he had taken *atropa-belladonna,* as he had a remarkably dilated pupil, and was frequently catching at objects, and his pulse was much accelerated, his face congested, and he was somewhat comatose. . . . I made him vomit, and from twelve to a score of the *atropa-belladonna* came from his stomach" (*OB,* Sept. 1846: pp. 744–47).

HYDROCYANIC ACID

Hydrocyanic acid—also called prussic acid and oil of almonds—and its salts occur in various plants and were prepared commercially. They are among the most rapid and deadly of poisons. Woodman and Tidy's textbook of forensic medicine astutely remarks that "very probably the vessel out of which the poison was taken in a case of suicide will be found near the person, or at any rate at no great distance off, the absence of the glass or bottle being always suggestive of homicide" (1877: p. 404). Tests for the acid and its salts were known in Christison's day (Christison, 1845: pp. 577–81). Surprisingly, in minute amounts prussic acid was used medicinally.

Water distilled from the cherry laurel, *Cerasus lauro-cerasus,* contains hydrocyanic acid. This liquid gained prominence during a fa-

33. Nettle berries do not exist. Whortleberries, also known as bilberries, blueberries, or huckleberries, somewhat resemble the fruit of belladonna (Bianchini and Corbetta, 1977: p. 136; Stuart, 1979: pp. 161, 277).

mous poisoning trial held in 1781, not at the Old Bailey but at the Warwick Assizes. The murder victim, Sir Theodosius Boughton, aged twenty and unmarried, would soon have come into an estate of about £2,000 a year. He lived at the family home with his mother, sister, and the latter's husband, Captain John Donellan. If Sir Theodosius were to die before he reached the age of twenty-one, most of the fortune he was to have inherited would go instead to his sister. The young man appeared to be in good health except for a "slight" venereal disease for which he was under treatment. Nevertheless, he often complained of not feeling well, an attitude which Donellan, his brother-in-law, seems to have encouraged.

Late on Tuesday afternoon, 29 August 1780, Sir Theodosius swallowed some of the draft sent to him by the local apothecary; it consisted of lavender water, nutmeg, jalap,[34] syrup of saffron, and water. This concoction was for the treatment of his venereal disease; the bottle was tactfully labeled "Purging draught for Sir Theodosius Boughton." He took more of the medicine, which was kept on an easily accessible shelf outside his bedroom, that evening. The next morning, when his mother came to give him a further dose, he complained of its nauseating taste and smell, "like bitter almonds." Nevertheless he swallowed what was left in the bottle. In a minute or two, the mother later testified, he struggled convulsively "and made a prodigious rattling in his throat and stomach, and a gurgling, and seemed to make very great efforts to keep it down." Within fifteen minutes his teeth were clenched, his eyes were fixed, and he frothed at the mouth. The apothecary, Mr. Powell, was sent for.

At this point Donellan came into the room and the mother exclaimed that she had given her son something that the apothecary must have sent in error. Donellan seized the medicine bottle, poured water into it, shook it, and emptied it into a hand basin containing dirty water. Next he ordered a woman servant to remove both bottle and basin, managing all this over Lady Boughton's objections. About this time Sir Theodosius died.

A few days later, largely at the urging of the dead man's guardian, an autopsy was called for. Donellan contrived various delays, and the corpse was not exhumed and opened until ten days after death had occurred. Then an inquest was ordered. Donellan wrote to the coroner that the dead man had kept arsenic about to kill rats and that he used it carelessly. Two physicians, a surgeon, and an Oxford anatomist offered testimony at the inquest. They agreed that Boughton had

34. A cathartic obtained from the root of the plant *Exogonium purga*.

died in consequence of drinking the draft, that the latter contained poison, and that the appearance of the body at autopsy resembled that of animals dead of poison. The coroner's jury indicted Donellan for wilful murder.

Stephen, an eminent legal historian, has stated that "the way in which they [the expert witnesses] were allowed to give their opinions differed much from what would be permitted in the present day, as their answers embodied their view of the evidence, with their opinion of the nature of the symptoms described. In the present day great pains are taken to prevent this, and to oblige skilled witnesses to give scientific opinions only, leaving the evidence to the jury" (1883: p. 382).

The trial was held on 30 March 1781. A good deal of circumstantial evidence was brought forward, as was the fact that Donellan possessed a still that could have been used to produce laurel water. Medical evidence for the prosecution was to the effect that the post-mortem findings were like those due to poison and that the latter was probably laurel water.

The chief expert witness for the defense was the renowned John Hunter. He had not participated in the autopsy but had been in court to hear the testimony of the medical men who had made the examination. They had conceded that they had not opened the head or intestines, even though the latter appeared to be inflamed. Hunter objected vigorously to such a delayed and incomplete examination and emphasized that the symptoms could have been occasioned either by poison or by cerebral hemorrhage. "The whole appearances upon the dissection explain nothing but putrefaction. . . . I should rather suspect it to be an apoplexy, and I wish the head had been opened. It might have removed all doubts." Under questioning by counsel, the doughty Scot added that he himself had dissected some thousands of bodies and had poisoned numerous dogs with laurel water. "I have injected laurel-water directly into the blood of dogs, and they have not died; I have thrown laurel-water, with a precaution, into the stomach, and it never produced so quick an effect with me, as described by those gentlemen." However, he had to admit to little experience with the effects of prussic acid.

Summing up, the judge, Mr. Justice Buller, after reviewing the evidence of the four expert witnesses for the prosecution, had this to say about John Hunter's refusal to commit himself beyond the bounds of the evidence:

> For the prisoner you have had one gentleman called, and a very able man. I can hardly say what his opinion is, for he does not seem to have formed any opinion at all of the matter. He, at first, said he could

> not form an opinion whether the death was, or was not, occasioned by the poison, because he could conceive that it might be ascribed to other causes. I wished, very much, to have got a direct answer from Mr. Hunter, if I could, what, upon the whole, was now the result of his attention and application to the subject; and what was his present opinion; but he says he can say nothing decisive. So that, upon this point, if you are to determine upon the evidence of the gentlemen who are skilled in the faculty only [the other medical experts], you have the very positive opinion, of four or five gentlemen of the faculty, that the deceased did die of poison. On the other side, you have what I really cannot myself call more than the doubt of another; for it is agreed, by Mr. Hunter, that the laurel-water would produce the symptoms which are described. He says, an epilepsy or apoplexy would produce the same symptoms; but, as to an apoplexy, it is not likely to attack so young, and so thin a man as Sir Theodosius was; and, as to an epilepsy, the other witnesses tell you, they don't think the symptoms which have been spoken of, do shew that Sir Theodosius had any epilepsy at the time.

The jury needed only nine minutes to decide that Captain Donellan was guilty. He was hanged three days later.[35]

Hunter's interpretation of the evidence he heard may or may not have been correct, but one must admire his refusal to go beyond it in forming an opinion. The judge's summing-up of the medical testimony could scarcely have not prejudiced the jury against Donellan; on the other hand, the circumstantial evidence does seem to suggest his guilt. It is not surprising that controversy about the case continued for many years.

More than a century later, forensic chemistry had progressed to the point where hydrocyanic acid was readily detected, as in an alleged attempt at forcible poisoning:

> GEORGE WILLIAM WIGNER. I . . . am a Fellow of the Chemical Society and of the Society of Analysts—on Monday, 11th December, I received from constable Morgan this small phial, tied over with a piece of washleather secured with red tape and bearing the seal of the Woolwich [police] station. . . . the smaller vial contained, as it came to me, two or at most three drops of a liquid—on removing the cork there was a very perceptible smell of prussic acid. . . . I tested it in five different ways and I found prussic acid and nothing else. (*OB,* Jan. 1877: pp. 359–63)

35. J. G. Smith, 1825: pp. 180–88; Christison, 1845: pp. 607–08; Stephen, 1883: *3,* 371–78: Glaister, 1954: pp. 109–10; Dobson, 1969: pp. 220–22; Cornelius, 1978.

OXALIC ACID

Five of the six Old Bailey poisoning cases involving oxalic acid occurred between February 1845 and July 1846; in two of them the accused was the same woman. Quite possibly some of these poisoning attempts were in imitation of others described in the press.

Oxalates occur in the juices of rhubarb, wood sorrel, common dock, and certain other plants. Commercial oxalic acid, "acid of sugar," a white powder, was used extensively as a metal cleaner and a bleach by brass workers, bookbinders, and leather workers. In the home it was often employed to remove ink stains and to clean brass. Taylor remarked that cases of oxalic acid poisoning were usually accidents or suicides; because of the difficulty of concealing the bitter taste of the acid in food or drink, it was seldom administered with homicidal intent (1848: p. 205). If ingested in sufficient amount it is fatal.

A man accused of homicide testified that he and a woman friend had each swallowed oxalic acid in a suicide pact. He recovered, but she died. Oxalic acid was found in a tumbler from which he said he had drunk. A surgeon described the results of the post-mortem examination:

> I attribute her death to inflammation of the lining membrane of the stomach, and the whole of the intestines, particularly the small intestines—that could be produced by any acrid poison. . . . a dark thick fluid blood in the stomach, of the consistency of tar—I attribute all that to the poison. . . . I analyzed the contents of the stomach, but could detect no oxalic acid by any test—persons generally vomit very freely before death, and the blood would very likely, and does, decompose oxalic acid, and oxalic acid decomposes the blood, so that it is very difficult when oxalic acid is once mixed with blood to find it. (*OB*, June 1845: pp. 237–44)

One notes the failure, once again, to identify a poison in the victim's body by test.

CHLORAL HYDRATE

Chloral hydrate, sometimes incorrectly referred to as chloral, played a role in a bizarre affair in 1876 that resulted in the trial of William Kingston Vance and Ellen Snee "for unlawfully conspiring to kill and murder Ellen Snee." The latter had placed the following advertisement in the *Daily Telegraph* in February 1876:

> To medical men in need of money, or students well up in chemistry and anatomy. A gentleman engaged in an interesting experiment is willing to give liberal remuneration for professional assistance. Q. W., Post Office, Junction Road, Kentish Town, N.W.[36]

Shortly thereafter she received a response, which she answered on 20 February as follows:

> Dear Sir, I make no question you could be of service to me, the question is will you? The *solatium* [compensation] I offer is £100. The conditions these. I am tired of my life. I could do a great deal of good to a person I am interested in by leaving the world just now, and one way or another I am resolved to do so, but, if possible, I should prefer not to wound the feelings of the person who will gain most by my death by allowing it to be supposed voluntary. *Besides, the most merciful verdict of a coroner's jury will be sufficient to invalidate my will* [italics added]. Now, although I have some acquaintance with medicine and chemistry, I know of no drug or combination of drugs which would do this for me without risk of discovery. It is possible you may. . . . I am willing to allow time for experiments, have no objection to a personal interview, and will give any assurance of *bona fides* that may be thought necessary; I only request that this communication be considered strictly private.
>
> Yours faithfully, M. Q.
>
> Address to these initials, at the P.O., Junction Road, Kentish Town, N.W.

Mrs. Snee's ladylike request for technical information as to the most suitable way to commit suicide received a prompt and enthusiastic response from her correspondent, William Kingston Vance. He was a twenty-four-year-old medical student who had completed the curriculum and was serving as *locum tenens* to a surgeon, John Gordon Mannering, looking after the latter's patients and enjoying full access to the surgery with its store of drugs. On 23 February Vance wrote to "M. Q.," giving full professional attention to the medical aspects of the proposed demise:

> My dear Sir,—It occurs to me I may not have very clearly explained my suggested *Modus operandi*. . . . I must say there is risk of discovery with whatever mode of death; for the registrar requires notice of "cause of death" from medical attendant. Should this be not forth-

36. "Q. W.", and subsequently also "M. Q.", "M. V.", and "William Quarll," were all Mrs. Snee.

coming, an inquest, and in all cases of sudden decease, an inquest. . . . My plan is this: Sudden death allowed, or apparently suspicious death acknowledged, still a favourable [coroner's] verdict may be returned which in no way can invalidate a will made antecedent to death, probably many weeks. The peculiarity of my suggestion is that although the actual cause of death is found out, and that a narcotic, yet the verdict will be the most lenient, viz., "By misadventure," or as it is phrased sometimes more specifically "The deceased was in the habit of taking chloral, and died from an overdose incautiously administered by himself." I can arrange details to "square" with this. . . . Upon mature consideration, I know of no more feasible method. The cases of the poisoners, Pritchard and Palmer, both doctors, were ingenious, yet they were detected. They lived before these chloral times. As an anatomist and medical jurist, I altogether frown on any attempt to excite arterial rupture, &c., and am willing to adduce reasons. . . . If you adopt my theory we might arrange to meet, and then take leave of the subject. . . . Expecting a reply.—

Believe me, Sir, in confidence, yrs., W. K. V.—M. Q.

This Olympian pronouncement did not end the correspondence. The next missive to be offered in testimony at the Old Bailey was as follows:

To be called for, M. V., 149, Kentish Town Road, Post-office, N.W. April 9. Dear Sir,—I cannot thank you enough for the admirable way in which you have managed everything. . . . I am inclined to think that the chloral will be perfectly satisfactory. . . . Is a portion of it equal to six teaspoons full of the labelled bottle *quite certain* in its effect? If you can assure me of this I shall not want any other medium, except, perhaps, a drop or two of prussic acid in a tiny phial. . . . I shall be in the City early tomorrow, and will post your fee whole. . . . you will want it for your holiday, perhaps. Don't forget the bill. I can trust my niece to see it paid, but you may have to wait six months after the event.[37] This lovely weather has given me great desire to see one particular spot of country in the North for the last time. I think I shall start on Tuesday afternoon and give myself a week's holiday. . . .

Your's most faithfully, Wm. Quarll. . . .

Vance answered on 12 April:

Dear Sir,—I notified to P.O., K.T. Rd. (149), that I received your letter, Monday. . . . The prussic acid is quite ready for post, and as for the essence of peppermint, you will find some three or four drops sufficient to flavour, and neutralise odour. . . . My full name is William Kingston Vance. Let my address remain, 59 Euston Road,

37. While the deceased's estate was being settled.

> N.W. . . . take *two good tablespoons.* It might be a good plan, having abstracted *your dose, before swallowing,* to pour in some clear water, but not to *the extent of filling,* for if the solution were found very strong and undiluted, suspicion were aroused. You understand you may employ either bottle. . . . Whichever bottle you use, throw the other away, and let the bottle you employ be left on the mantelpiece or table, not by the bed. Let no specimen of my writing, save that relating to debt, be found; and let all around you remain in usual condition, to imply absence of design. The entire affair is to show *prima facie* accident.

Vance clearly had included forensic medicine in his professional studies.

At the trial Mr. Mannering, for whom this remarkable young man had been *locum tenens,* identified Vance's handwriting and spoke highly of his professional conduct. Another witness was a detective sergeant. For reasons that were not explained at the trial, the suspicions of the police regarding Mrs. Snee had been aroused, and the officer, John R. Manton, was instructed to watch her. Manton saw her make out a money order at a post office and receive various letters. Post Office employees identified her and also a money order for £2.2.0 signed "W. Quarll" and payable to Vance. Other witnesses identified a bottle labeled chloral that had been purchased from a firm of chemists and the draft of the original advertisement, brought to the *Daily Telegraph* for insertion in the paper on 16 February.

Thomas Bond, Fellow of the Royal College of Surgeons and Lecturer on Forensic Medicine at the Westminster Hospital, stated that the bottle offered in evidence contained what smelled like chloral and added that

> this bottle would contain equivalent to 1 oz. of solid chloral—to the best of my judgement and knowledge the half of it would cause death—the effect of a fatal dose of chloral is that the patient passes away and leaves no trace of having been poisoned, beyond the symptoms of coma and great sleep; we should not find anything upon a post-mortem examination to communicate the precise nature of the thing which had caused death, except by an analysis of the contents of the stomach, then it would be possible, if we analysed recently, by distillation to get the volatile particles of chloral. . . . it is very quickly absorbed, it would be impossible to find it except upon a very complete examination, shortly after death.

The prosecution nearly lost its case on points of law, counsel for the defense arguing that the relevant statute was "intended to apply to a conspiracy to murder a third person, and not one of the parties charged." It was also urged that the attempt to commit suicide did not constitute an attempt to commit murder, and was only a misdemeanor. The jury, however, found both of the accused to be guilty. Vance was sentenced to imprisonment for eighteen months; Mrs. Snee for six months (*OB,* May 1876: pp. 162–73; *Central,* 1876).

Discovery of the hypnotic action of chloral, announced to the medical profession only a few years earlier, had created much interest. Professional journals carried numerous articles and letters about both its virtues and its hazards (Earles, 1969). Vance seems to have been well informed about the drug. It was unfortunate that his medical ethics were not at the level of his intellect.

CHLOROFORM

The use of drugs to render a victim unconscious in order to simplify the commission of a crime was unusual but not unknown. Christison commented in 1845 regarding opium that "in recent times it has been made use of to commit murder, and to induce stupor previous to the commission of a robbery. . . . during the last fifteen years many persons have been brought into great danger by opium having been administered as a narcotic to facilitate robbery; and some have actually been killed" (1845: p. 530). Woodman and Tidy state that since unconsciousness is induced relatively slowly by chloroform, it "would be difficult . . . to administer chloroform to persons forcibly and against their will, whilst, of course, the stories of immediate anaesthesia are but idle fables" (1877: p. 457).

At an Old Bailey trial of two young women arrested for robbery, it was suggested that chloroform might have been used to overcome the victim, a young man named Jewett who allegedly was attacked on the street at night:

> I was perfectly sober, I had only a little claret—I felt someone at my left side—from a glance I had, I think it was a woman—I felt a handkerchief, or rag, come over my face, and have no idea of anything from that time till I found myself in a room on a horrible bed, naked, except my stockings. . . . there was no candle—I missed my boots, hat, a cashmere shawl, gloves, handkerchief, silver watch, hair-guard,[38] a tooth-pick, a gold ring, two shillings, and some coppers—I had them all the night before, the ring had been in my waistcoat pocket with my tooth-pick—my waistcoat was not gone—the room-door was fastened outside.

38. A watch chain made of hair.

A police officer testified that he had been following the two accused women, Margaret Higgins and Elizabeth Smith, known as Fat Bet. They lived in the house in a disreputable neighborhood where young Jewett had said he was robbed. Further statements from the witness box again give a glimpse of the London underworld.

Police Sergeant Thomas Kelly arrested Margaret Higgins:

> I told her she was charged with drugging and robbing a gentleman at 9, Thrall-street—she said, "*I* did not do it, *Fat Bet* brought him to my room; she robbed him of this things, *cut* with and *stuck* to the regulars, (meaning that she kept the money); God strike me blind if I get *lagged* any more than the other, as one was as much in it as the other; and if you go to Hart's house, in George-street, you will find her there tonight, or at *Irish Mog's,* (that is the girl of the town who lives next door), but you must not tell that *I* told you, or they will kill me when I come out.

John Johns, another policeman, told of the subsequent arrest of the second prisoner:

> I and another officer went to a house in George-street. . . . I went to the back-door, and my brother officer to the front—I heard a knock at the front door, and a male voice said, "So help me God, *Bill,* it is the *copper, hook it*"—*copper* means policeman, and *hook it,* make your escape—the back-door was opened from the inside, and Smith came out partly undressed—I knew her before by the name of *Fat Bet*—she tried to escape from the passage—I stopped her.

Following this instructive testimony Christopher Lerick, a surgeon, came to the witness stand. He stated:

> I attended Mr. Jewitt for jaundice five weeks previous to this outrage—I have heard his account, and believe his becoming insensible might have been occasioned by chloroform—from the state in which I found him, I think laudanum was given him after the chloroform—a person could not become insensible by having laudanum put to his nose. . . . He was not sick after I was called to him; but was in a state of stupor, and had a contracted pupil, a hard pulse, and giddiness—I believe the effects of chloroform go off speedily.

The prisoners were found guilty and each was sentenced to transportation for fifteen years (*OB,* Feb. 1850: pp. 423–25).

Stupor, pupillary contraction, and vomiting in the recovery phase are usual in nonfatal opium poisoning; it seems likely that Jewitt was drugged with laudanum administered in a drink of some kind. The surgeon produced no real evidence that chloroform had been used.

Sir James Y. Simpson, the distinguished Edinburgh obstetrician, introduced the use of chloroform for surgical anesthesia in November

1847 after becoming convinced that it was superior to ether as an anesthetic during deliveries (1847a, b). Chloroform quickly gained wide popularity with British medical men in spite of a good many fatal accidents associated with its use (Mettler, 1947: p. 220). Along with public acclaim for the new anesthetic grew the fear that it could be employed to induce instant unconsciousness when a robbery or other crime was to be committed, a false idea shared by some members of the medical profession. John Snow,[39] a prominent London anesthetist, was sufficiently disturbed by this error to send a lengthy letter of correction to the *London Medical Gazette* on 13 February 1850, just after the trial of Smith and Higgins:

> I cannot explain how the prosecutor [Jewitt] got to the room of the prisoners, but I wish to state very distinctly my conviction that it was not by means of chloroform, and that, if anything was administered on a handkerchief in Whitechapel, it must have been some agent unknown to medical men, and which, if the police could discover it, would probably be of great service to humanity in the hands of legitimate practitioners. (Snow, 1850; Mason, 1980)

In summary, one is struck with the easy availability and relatively frequent homicidal use of arsenic and opium. The statistician William Farr, well aware of the problem, wrote bitterly of "poisons, which can be procured of the most subtle and destructive nature, with extraordinary facility" (1840: p. 77). The great forensic medical problem was the overwhelming necessity for the expert witness to be able to prove that a lethal amount of a particular poison had been administered. Sometimes a significant residue could be demonstrated, if uncertainly, in organs and body fluids, although, as Alfred Swaine Taylor pointed out, it is not the poison *in* the digestive tract but that which has been *absorbed* that kills. Toxicology was still a young science; a grasp of Orfila's contributions on the Continent seems to have come slowly to British medical men. Except for the Marsh test for arsenic, reliable procedures for identification and measurement of poisons were yet to appear.

39. This physician (1813–58) had introduced into Britain in 1847 a method for the controlled administration of ether during surgery (Snow, 1847; Inhalation, 1847). He is better known for his dramatic demonstration that drinking water contaminated with sewage transmitted cholera.

IX

Insanity

The boundaries of sanity and insanity are very ill-defined—it is a most difficult task to express a scientific opinion as to the state of a man's brain.

John Rowland Gibson,
Surgeon of Newgate Gaol
(OB, Dec. 1876: p. 259)

FORENSIC PSYCHIATRY DIFFERED FROM OTHER AREAS OF FORENSIC MEDICINE in being concerned not only with fact but with large areas of uncertainty and hence of interpretation and controversy. When the medical man and the barrister, each accustomed to precise definitions, to specifics, to tangible problems, confronted the case of a mentally disturbed individual accused of a crime, they entered on a path that began on firm ground but soon entered a morass with scanty and none too visible stepping stones. Proof that an offense had been *committed* by the accused was usually solid enough; it was the definition and determination of his or her legal *responsibility* and "guilt" that often ended in a quagmire of confusion and conflict. Yet this was the only route toward protection of the individual, of society, and of justice. In the following examination of a large and difficult field, we shall have glimpses of how the morass and the paths developed.[1]

1. Particularly valuable sources of information included books and articles by Biggs, 1955; Jones, 1955; Dreher, 1967; Walker, 1968; Lewinstein, 1969; Allderidge, 1974; Quen, 1974; R. Smith, 1981.

Since this book is concerned with forensic medicine in the criminal but not the civil court, we shall not consider the responsibilities of the medical man in civil actions, for example, in questions of mental competence to sign a will, to enter into a contract, or to marry.

The term *insanity* at present usually refers to mental illness but not to mental defectiveness such as idiocy. Although the word *insane* was in use as early as the sixteenth century, it seems to have had little vogue until the late 1800s. Much more common was *lunatic,* employed in various connotations and defined in the 1845 Lunatics Act as meaning "every insane person, and every person being an idiot or lunatic or of unsound mind" (K. Jones, 1955: p. x).

In this chapter we shall see how insanity came to be recognized as possible exculpation for an offense, how a distinction arose between complete and partial insanity, and how repeated attempts were made both to define and to determine the degrees and kinds of insanity which would relieve an accused person of legal guilt for his harmful act. By necessity, the definitions and tests and their interpretation began their evolution in the courts, which in time turned to medical experts for assistance, and gradually the opinions of forensic psychiatrists came to be recognized as of crucial importance. If in the process definitions of "not guilty by reason of insanity" were partly clarified, they were scarcely simplified. The situation was not helped when forensic medical experts for the defense differed with those for the prosecution. The problem continues today.

Dreher explains how in the seventh century there arose in English law what might be termed the theory of *absolute liability,* which stated that lack of guilt, accident, lunacy, or infancy did *not* excuse a criminal act. In the same century there emerged the Canon Law of the Church, defining the circumstances that imputed *moral* guilt. Much later, partly due to the influence of Henry de Bracton (died 1268), a cleric who served as judge in both secular and ecclesiastical courts, the religious concept of moral guilt entered criminal law to modify and replace the theory of absolute liability. "This moral guilt," says Dreher, "took the form of *blame,* or sin, and these terms came, in time, to mean *intent* or *mens rea*" ("guilty mind"). According to Bracton, for homicide to be considered a crime the act must be coupled with an intent or will to injure. The act and the intent together thus constituted criminal responsibility (Dreher, 1967: pp. 49–52; Biggs, 1955: pp. 81–83). Bracton did not believe that an insane person should be considered liable for his or her offense (Lewinstein, 1969).

As previously suggested, in undertaking the "insanity defense" of an accused person, the chief difficulty arose not in proving that the accused had committed the offense but in defining and determining his *intent* to injure. This situation, incidentally, is in interesting contrast to the defense of a sane person accused of homicide, where proof of *commission* of the crime by the accused is likely to be the chief problem of the prosecution.

William Lambarde (1536–1601), legal and general historian, lawyer, and archivist, was also a justice of the peace for Kent. In his book *Eirenarcha,* first published in 1581, which dealt with the duties of justices of the peace, he specified the four kinds of persons not to be punished for a homicide, since the law denied that they had "a will, or mind to doe the harme, as a madde man, he that is borne both deafe and dumbe, nor an infant under the age of 12. yeres, unlesse it may be some evident token appeare that he had understanding of good and evill, for then in him *Malicia supplebit aetatem* ["malice will make up for age"], and to these (by the opinion of M[aster] Bracton) you may add the Lunatike during that disease for a fourth" (1602: bk. 2, chap. 7, p. 236). The phrase "Lunatike during that disease" reflects the contemporary idea that lunacy was a transitory condition. We note also the essential reference to "understanding of good and evil," a corollary to the concept of moral guilt.

Inevitably, the issue of whether an insane person could be responsible for a felony came to be tested in court. No doubt such cases occurred as early as Bracton's time, but the first written record of an English medical man appearing in the role of what would now be called a forensic psychiatrist seems to be that of Edward Jorden. In 1602 he testified in defense of Elizabeth Jackson, an old woman on trial for having bewitched Mary Glover, aged fourteen, causing her to suffer from dreadful fits and temporary speechlessness, blindness, paralysis, and other afflictions. On the witness stand the physicians who had treated Mary without success ascribed her condition to "some cause beyond naturall," that is, witchcraft. Jorden and Dr. John Argent[2] testified that Mary's illness was due to natural causes arising from the "mother" or uterus, but Elizabeth Jackson was found guilty. The trial impelled Jorden to write a book on the uterine origin of hysteria. Its lengthy but explanatory title was *A Briefe discourse of a disease called suffocation of the mother. Written upon occasion which hath beene of late taken thereby, to suspect possession of an evill spirit, or some such like supernaturall power. Wherein is declared that divers strange actions and passions of the body of man, which in the common opinion, are imputed to the*

2. Argent (died 1643) was later to be the friend of William Harvey and eight times President of the Royal College of Physicians.

Divell, have their true naturall causes, and do accompanie this disease (1603). As Hunter and Macalpine point out, the case was notable not only for Jorden's defense but because even at this early time "expert medical witnesses were called on both sides and disagreed fundamentally on a psychiatric issue" (1963: p. 70).

In 1628 the jurist Edward Coke, commenting on a treatise by Sir Thomas Littleton (1422–81), outlined four classes of the condition *non compos mentis* ("not having control of the mind," insane): he who "from his nativitie, by a perpetuall infirmitie," is an idiot, "Hee that by sicknesse, griefe, or other accident, wholly loseth his memorie and understanding. 3. a lunatique that hath sometimes his understanding and sometimes not . . . and therefore he is called *non compos mentis*, so long as he hath not understanding. Lastly, hee that by his owne vitious act for a time depriveth himselfe of his memorie and understanding, as he that is drunken" (1794: sect. [247a]; Quen, 1974). Here a lack of "understanding" is the essential characteristic of the lunatic. But as Lewinstein (1969: p. 276) observes, Coke did not define the *degree* of lack of understanding which must exist in order to avoid criminal responsibility.

Lord Matthew Hale, another distinguished judge, did attempt such a definition:

> Man is naturally endowed with these two great faculties, understanding and liberty of will . . . . The consent of the will is that, which renders human actions either commendable or culpable; as where there is no law, there is no transgression, so regularly, where there is no will to commit an offense, there can be no transgression. . . . And because the liberty of choice of the will presupposeth an act of the understanding to know the thing or action chosen by the will, it follows that where there is a total defect of the understanding, there is no free act of the will in the choice of things or actions.

Recognizing that, while insanity may be "total" or partial, only the former presupposes lack of criminal intent, Hale defines sanity. "The best measure that I can think of is this: such a person as labouring under melancholy distempers hath yet ordinarily as great understanding as ordinarily a child of fourteen years hath, is such a person as may be guilty of treason, or felony" (1736: 1, pp. 14–16).

LAY DETERMINATION OF INSANITY

Twelve years before Hale's *Historia placitorum coronae,* from which the foregoing is quoted, was published posthumously in 1736, Edward

Arnold was brought to trial for shooting Lord Onslow with intent to kill. The nobleman was wounded, but not fatally. Judge Robert Tracy, instructing the jury as to the mental state of the accused, stated that the question was

> whether this man hath the use of his reason and sense? If he . . . could not distinguish between good and evil, and did not know what he did . . . he could not be guilty of any offense against any law whatsoever . . . . On the other side . . . it is not every kind of frantic humour or something unaccountable in a man's actions that points him out to be such a madman as to be exempted from punishment; it must be a man that is *totally* deprived of his understanding and memory, and doth not know what he is doing, no more than an infant, than a brute, or wild beast;[3] such a one is never the object of punishment. (quoted by Walker, 1968: p. 56)

Sentenced to the gallows, Arnold was saved by the intervention of Lord Onslow but spent the rest of his life behind bars.

More than a century after the trial the American psychiatrist Isaac Ray commented, "It appears, then, that the law at that time did not consider an insane person irresponsible for crime, in whom there remained the slightest degree of rationality" (1838: pp. 16–19). Arnold seems to have been dangerously psychotic but to have retained a degree of sanity (Biggs, 1955: p. 88). Dreher has cogently remarked that in effect Judge Tracey was stating that "proof of insanity established lack of intent." Not resolved were the continuing problems of "the *nature* of the insanity that prevents the formation of the required intent" (Dreher, 1967: p. 53) and, as a corollary, a satisfactory test for such insanity.

In 1730 Peter Bluck sought out a justice of the peace and told him that two and a half years earlier he, Bluck, had murdered his five-year-old daughter. The father was arraigned and pleaded guilty, "but the Court being credibly inform'd that the Prisoner was not in his right Mind, and perceiving some Token of Distraction in him at the Bar, refus'd to take his Plea; but the next Day being brought to the Bar, and pleading not Guilty, the Court proceeded to examine the Witnesses for the King."

First among these was the justice mentioned above, who deposed that the prisoner said his conscience had moved him to confess the murder. Bluck had told the justice how he had hanged his daughter, then cut her down and sent for an apothecary, pretending that the

3. Italics added. Tracey's dictum gave rise to what became known as the "wild beast test" (Lodge, 1901: p. 53).

child had had an apoplectic fit. The apothecary, finding that the child was dead and observing, he said, no marks of violence, accepted the father's story, as did a parish searcher. "Another witness deposed that Bluck had several times given a Guinea a time to a Minister to pray by him, and had given away 400 ℓ in five Weeks time, and had scarce a Six Pence left to help himself; there being no Evidence against the Prisoner, but his own Confession, the Jury acquitted him" (*OB*, July 1730: pp. 12–13).

One assumes that the apothecary and the searcher, feeling sorry for Bluck, simply failed to report what must have been the obvious signs of strangulation. There were no other expert witnesses. The court made no recommendation regarding Bluck's future.

The following year Edward Stafford, brother of Lord Stafford, was tried for fatally wounding Thomas Mainwaring with a sword before a witness. At the trial there was again no medical testimony except as to the fatal injuries. But numerous lay witnesses described the delusions and bizarre actions of the accused, who clearly was what would now be termed paranoid. Lord Stafford deposed that he had sought a medical man to commit Edward to confinement; however, there was a delay, and the assault occurred. The jury brought in a verdict of lunacy (*OB,* July 1731: pp. 11–16; Walker, 1968: pp. 57–58). This time the decision as to the sanity of the accused was entirely in the hands of laymen.

In a subsequent case, when a man indicted for murder was brought to trial, "His appearance at the bar seeming to discover he was not right in his senses, the following evidences were sworn, for the Middlesex jury to determine whether he was, or was not of sound mind and memory, fit to take his trial, &c." In this interesting departure from the usual court procedure, what we would call a sanity hearing was conducted *preliminary* to trial. All the witnesses again apparently were laymen. The prisoner had lodged with one of them, William Nichols, who concluded that the accused was "not in his senses." Nichols saw him again in New Prison:

> *Q.* How was his state of mind then?
> *Nichols.* In a very indifferent manner, very bad . . . .
> *Q.* As to his behaviour since he has been in prison, do you think it was counterfeit or real?
> *Nichols.* Really, my lord, it is real.
> *Court.* People that counterfeit are very often off their guard; did you see anything that could induce you to believe that it was put on?
> *Nichols.* It was real I am sure.

The jury found the man not of sound mind and memory (*OB*, June 1756: pp. 233–34; Walker, 1968: pp. 222–23). Decades later Forbes Winslow was to comment regarding the simulation of lunacy that the "person who is desirous of appearing insane, generally exhibits his sanity by overacting the part of a madman. The real maniac, although known to be deranged, will often absolutely deny that he is so" (1843: p. 77).

The disposition of prisoners found to be insane was not specified in the court records at this period. If the individual were confined, it might be as a pauper lunatic under the jurisdiction of the parish overseer, in a prison, in a private madhouse (Parry-Jones, 1973), in Bethlehem Hospital, an institution for the acutely insane, or in a private house, with or without medical attendance. Custodial treatment ranged from sympathetic attention to, more commonly, abuse, neglect, and confinement in chains or a cell (Jones, 1955: pp. 9–11, 31–37; Walker and McCabe, 1968: 2, 1–2).

The doctor in the eighteenth century was moving very slowly toward the medicolegal arena. William Battie's *A Treatise on Madness*, appeared in 1758. Instead of seeing lunacy as due to "vitiated judgment," he viewed it as a delusion of the imagination. He emphasized careful study of the individual patient before undertaking his treatment, which Battie believed should be adjusted to the needs of the individual. The reformer's criticisms evoked a spirited response from John Monro, physician at Bethlehem Hospital, entitled *Remarks on Dr. Battie's Treatise on Madness* (1758). Monro disagreed wholeheartedly with Battie. The controversy did much to attract the attention of the public and the medical profession to problems of the insane (Hunter and Macalpine, 1962: pp. 13–17).

Then Francis David Stirn, a German, came to trial at the Old Bailey in September 1760 for the fatal shooting of Richard Mathews. Samuel Chapman, a surgeon and an acquaintance of Stirn, was put on the stand:

> Q. Did you ever see any signs of insanity by him?
> *Chapman*. Sometimes his behaviour has been very extraordinary, that I could not account for.
> Q. Do you think he was curable by medicine of this flighty madness?
> *Chapman*. I can't say.
> Q. Do you think he was mad enough to be put into Bedlam?
> *Chapman*. I believe not . . . .He appeared to be strangely agitated, but I can't pretend to say that it was madness.

Chapman and others then described several suicidal attempts Stirn had made as well as another assault he had committed.

The jury took only one minute to decide that Stirn was guilty. Sentenced to be hanged, he took poison in his cell and was "buried in a cross road, with a stake through him, near Black Mary's Hole" (*OB*, Sept. 1760: pp. 262–74). The law required that a suicide, unless deranged, be buried at night and in this barbarous manner (Forbes, 1971: pp. 165–69).

It is unfortunate that the *Sessions Papers* do not include the judge's summing-up in the Stirn trial. We might have been given some clues as to the legal basis on which guilt was determined. It is evident, however, that in this case what Chapman called "periodical madness" did not absolve Stirn from the guilt of homicide either of another or of himself.

More notorious was the murder in the same year by Earl Ferrers of his factor. As a nobleman, Ferrers was tried by his peers with full ceremony in the House of Lords in April 1760. There was little doubt of the facts, and presentation of the Crown's case was brief. Under the law, Ferrers was obliged to conduct his own defense. Among those he called was Dr. John Monro. According to Winslow (1843: p. 26), testimony included the allegation that insanity was hereditary in Ferrers's family. The test of insanity, in Dreher's words, "was held to be the ability to distinguish between good and evil generally, or in the abstract, rather than with respect to the particular act charged" (1967: p. 53). In yet another instance of lay judgment of sanity, Ferrers was found guilty by unanimous vote of his peers and was hanged at Tyburn.[4]

Now came a much more penetrating attempt by a layman, this time a judge, to evaluate the mental state of a prisoner. William Walker, in the ancient words of the murder charge, "not having the fear of God before his eyes, but being moved and seduced by the instigation of the Devil," was indicted in 1784 for killing his wife Ann with a clasp knife. Walker was a day laborer. The friends and neighbors who were asked to testify about his mental state seem to have been reluctant to give evidence of his unusual behavior, although one or two, including the constable who arrested him, did say that at times he was "troubled." In a lengthy charge to the jury, the perceptive and distinguished

4. Winslow, 1843: pp. 25–27; Biggs, 1955: pp. 91–92; Walker, 1968: pp. 55–63; Lewinstein, 1969: p. 278.

judge, Mr. Baron Eyre (1734–99), first pointed out that there was no doubt that Walker had killed his wife. The Court continued,

> unless it is established in his favour, that he did this under such an impression, and in such a state of mind that ought not to make him answerable for what he has done, unquestionably he is guilty of the crime of wilful murder imputed to him . . . . the whole case is brought to turn upon a single point, whether this man, at the time he committed this outrage upon his wife, was in his right mind or no, whether he did it from motives of wickedness and malice toward her, or whether he did it under the impression of some distemper of mind which had deprived him of the use of his reason . . . . if you should really see reason to collect from the evidence, that at the moment he committed the act, he was not in possession of himself, that he was not in possession of his right senses, and of his right mind, but that it was done under the pressure of some disorder of mind, occasioned by something that you and I cannot get to the bottom of, that will make him nothing more than a mere instrument in the hands of Providence . . . . it appears to me, that this [murder] was the unhappy effect of rage against this woman, conceived in consequence of distemper of mind, brought on by disease, and that under the impression the violence was committed. The man's afterwards coming to his senses will not alter the nature of the case, if it was committed under the impression of insanity . . . . Indeed he is either guilty of the crime of wilful murder, or he is a mere machine.

The jury brought in a verdict of not guilty. Thereupon the court ordered: "This man must not be discharged, unless the parish officers, to save the expences, come and take him away [to confinement]; he must be carried before a magistrate, confined, and taken proper care of" (*OB,* Mar. 1784: pp. 529–49).

Mr. Baron Eyre took a similarly enlightened position in his remarks from the bench at the trial of John Simpson, who stabbed his wife fatally during what was interpreted as an attack of temporary insanity. The judge stated that he was satisfied that the insanity was genuine and not simulated, and advised the jury to find the prisoner not guilty. The jury decided accordingly, and recommended that Simpson "be taken care of." The court expressed the hope that his friends would find a way to do so (*OB,* April 1786: pp. 584–603).

Another issue that arose was, not surprisingly, that of the relation of drunkenness to mental imbalance. James Carse, a sailor, found himself in the dock at the Old Bailey in 1787 because while intoxicated he had fatally wounded his wife with a clasp knife. The assault was admitted by the prisoner. Carse was alleged to conduct himself in a normal way except when he was drunk. Expert medical testimony would have been appropriate, but the principal witness in his defense was Horatio Nelson, not yet an admiral, under whom Carse had served in the frigate *Boreas:*

> *Mr. Garrow to Captain Nelson.* Had you an opportunity of knowing the character of this man, as far as humanity and good-nature were concerned?—Perfectly . . . . he appeared to me to be a man that had seen better days, and at times became melancholy; when I heard of this affair, I said, if it is true, he must be insane, for I should as soon suspect myself . . . . seamen, I know perfectly, when they come home, the landlords will furnish them with raw liquors; I saw myself thirty or forty people from that ship, that were made as mad as if they were at Bedlam, and did not know what they did; I know, that when seamen are furnished with British spirits, it turns the brain.

The judge, Mr. Justice Heath, instructing the jury, declared that

> The excuse here is madness; if that excuse has been proved to the utmost of its extent, and to your satisfaction, it would undoubtedly be a reasonable one, but then the madness that is brought on a prisoner, must arise from the visitation of God; it must be the consequences of some disease; but even if there be antecedent disease, if there be the seeds of madness lurking in the blood, and the party be reasonable and in his senses, in the ordinary transactions of life, and he voluntarily inflames his blood, and by means of drunkenness, draws out that madness which before was lurking in it, the law does not excuse him . . . . it seems pretty clear, that at the time he committed this act, he clearly was mad . . . . if you think that when he was sober and free from liquor, he knew what he was about, and was capable of discerning right from wrong (and the captain tells you he was) then it is no excuse at all that he got drunk.

The jury found him guilty (*OB,* Dec. 1787: pp. 5–12).

Insanity as a medicolegal problem was recalled dramatically to public attention when attempts were made on the life of royalty. George III, himself in a precarious mental state (Macalpine and Hunter, 1969), was the victim of attacks by unbalanced persons. On 2 August 1786 a servant, Margaret Nicholson, tried to stab him with a dessert knife. Following her arrest, the king intervened, requesting humane treatment for the prisoner. Investigations by the Privy Council and by Dr. Thomas Monro, like his father, John, physican to Bethlehem Hospital, resulted in a verdict of insanity and in an order from the Secretary of State that the woman be permanently confined.[5]

On 21 January 1790, while George III was being driven in a state procession to attend the House of Lords, John Frith, dressed in a

5. K. Jones, 1955: p. 204; Walker, 1968: pp. 185–86; Allderidge, 1974.

bizarre costume, threw a stone at the coach. He was arrested, interrogated at some length, and placed in prison, where he was examined by a physician of the king. On 17 April Frith came to trial for high treason. This charge entitled him to defense counsel; he was represented by Mr. Shepherd and Mr. Garrow. They requested postponement of the trial so that "some very important evidence" could be procured. To this the prosecution agreed and Frith disagreed. After argument, the court directed that the jury should then and there investigate Frith's present sanity. So the jury members were sworn to "diligently enquire . . . whether John Frith . . . be of sound mind and understanding," attention, significantly, being directed toward his mental state not at the time of the attack but at that of the trial.

Frith thereupon entered into a lengthy defense, prompted by occasional questions by counsel. At first he seemed rational, making reference, incidentally, to Dr. William Heberden (1710–1801), one of the most distinguished physicians of his day, who had attended both Frith and his father. Before long, however, the prisoner spoke of a visit to Liverpool, where "I perceived I had some powers like those which St. Paul had; and the sun that St. Paul gives a description of in the Testament; and extraordinary power that came down upon me, the power of Christ . . . . when I came to London to the king concerning some military business, I told him nothing about any supernatural powers, or the power of God." Four laymen then testified that they had had repeated contact with the prisoner and believed him to be insane, one of them also quoting a Dr. Millan to the same effect. The jury unanimously concluded that Frith was "quite insane," and he was remanded. Here the court record ends (*OB,* April 1790: pp. 359–66; Walker, 1968: pp. 186, 223–24).

MEDICAL CERTIFICATION

Robert Natcot was brought to trial at the Old Bailey in 1790 for causing the death of Moses Davis by striking him on the head with a large iron key. Natcot had earlier been confined in Bedlam. At the trial there was medical testimony about the victim's injuries and the fact that Natcot was considered to be deranged. Then a Mr. Barney, a surgeon, deposed that he had treated a wound on Natcot's leg sixteen days before the attack on Davis. Said Barney:

> from his mode of behaviour, from his conversation, and in a word, the whole line of his conduct . . . I judged him at that time a lunatic: I

> continued to see him daily from that time. . . . when I found there was no doing anything with him, and that he was a dangerous man to society, I recommended him to be got into St. Luke's: and till then to be conveyed to Mr. Harrison's private mad-house: that I would fill up certificates, and get a friend in town[6] to sign them . . . . the certificates were, that in my judgment he was a lunatic.

Barney added that he again saw Natcot the day before the attack and urged his confinement as a dangerous person. On the direction of the judge, the jury found the prisoner not guilty by reason of insanity (*OB*, Sept. 1790: pp. 796–99).

This seems to be the first mention in the *Sessions Papers* of medical certification of insanity, although professional certification of private mental patients had been specified in the 1774 Madhouse Act in the effort to prevent confinement of the *sane* (Scull, 1979: p. 151), an abuse by no means unknown at the time.

THE HADFIELD CASE

The case of James Hadfield has been discussed repeatedly and at length.[7] A loyal and courageous dragoon, Hadfield received severe head injuries in battle in France in 1794. Suffering thereafter from periodic attacks of insanity, he was discharged from the army. At times he believed he was King George. Ackerknecht and Kozelka describe Hadfield as schizophrenic (1950: p. 1302). Entertaining the delusion that by giving his own life he could prevent God's destruction of the world, but not wishing to commit suicide, Hadfield decided to shoot King George III so as to ensure execution as a regicide (Quen, 1974). On 15 May 1800 the lunatic fired a loaded pistol at the monarch at Drury Lane Theatre but missed. Having failed to kill the king, the assailant was indicted not for murder but for high treason.

At his trial he was defended by the brilliant attorney Thomas Erskine, later to become Lord Chancellor. Erskine questioned the theory, proposed at the trials of Lord Ferrers and others, that only a total loss of memory freed an individual from criminal responsibility for his wrongful act. Alternatively, Erskine argued, the presence of delusions might obviate such responsibility. "Delusion, therefore,

6. Barney lived in Sudbury, about thirty-five miles from London.

7. Lodge, 1901; Ackerknecht and Kozelka, 1950: p. 1302; Biggs, 1955: pp. 88–90; Jones, 1955: pp. 204–05; Walker, 1968: pp. 74–81; Lewinstein, 1969: pp. 278–79; Quen, 1969, 1974; Allderidge, 1974; Ormrod, 1977: p. 5; R. Smith 1981: p. 20.

where there is no frenzy or raving madness is the true character of insanity" (quoted by Lewinstein, 1969: p. 279). That Hadfield was indeed mad was argued at some length both by Erskine and by an expert witness, a Dr. "Creighton" from Bethlehem Hospital,[8] who shortly before the trial had examined Hadfield for perhaps half an hour. Hadfield's mental state having been established by the testimony, Erskine suggested that the trial be terminated. The Attorney General agreed, and the Lord Chief Justice stopped the proceedings. The court thereupon virtually directed the jury to bring in a verdict of not guilty, the accused "being under the influence of insanity at the time the act was committed" (quoted by Biggs, 1955: p. 90).

Hadfield could either be continued illegally in custody—he had now been acquitted—or be released with the knowledge that he was dangerous to society. It became evident that a change in the law was needed, and within a month there was passed the Criminal Lunatics Act (40 Geo. 3, c. 94), which made possible a verdict of not guilty by reason of insanity and provided for the safe custody at His Majesty's pleasure of persons on whom this verdict was pronounced. Hadfield remained in confinement.

Public interest in the Hadfield case encouraged the physician John Johnstone (1768–1836) to publish his *On Madness* (1800). In it he discussed, among other topics, the extent to which lunacy may be due to heredity and to family environment. "Madness," he said, "can only be deemed an hereditary disease, insomuch, as children have a structure similar to that of their parents who have been mad, and as this peculiar organization is likely to be acted upon by the peculiar manners and habits of the parent in education" (p. 46). Johnstone believed that insanity may be produced by disease, anxiety, excess of drink, venery, fevers, and the post-partum period, a state which "is probably occasioned by organic laesion, and its duration is proportional to the injury sustained" (pp. 16–17; Hunter and Macalpine, 1963: p. 576).

THE INSANITY DEFENSE

What has come to be called "the insanity defense" was employed on a good many occasions at the Old Bailey during the nineteenth century. Concurrently there emerged the figure of what we would call the

8. This was probably Alexander Crichton, an alienist.

forensic psychiatrist. Although his testimony was clearly important and carried weight with a jury, he was not invariably summoned to the witness box in the trial of a mentally disturbed prisoner. Sometimes the judge took it on himself to deal with the question of sanity. For example, when John Nardi and Sebastian Grandi were tried for a murder, a physician, Dr. Simmons, gave it as his opinion that Nardi was a "deranged man" at the time of the assault and also of the trial. Charging the jury, the judge, Mr. Baron Graham, concluded: "Gentlemen, you will give me your verdict whether you are perfectly satisfied that Nardi was deranged in his mind at the time he committed this act or not; you will say whether the prisoner Nardi did this act of murder or no, or whether the prisoner Nardi was insane at the time he did this act. If you are of that opinion you will say so." The jury found him insane when he killed his victim, and it was directed that he "be kept in custody until His Majesty's pleasure shall be known" (*OB,* Dec. 1806: pp. 25–34). It is of interest that the judge speaks not of a degree of insanity but rather of whether insanity was present.

Another criterion, the "right and wrong test," emerged again at the trial of John Bellingham. This individual, who clearly suffered from paranoia, was convinced that the British government owed him a large sum of money. On Monday, 11 May 1812, in the House of Commons he shot and killed Sir Spencer Perceval, First Lord of the Exchequer, with a pistol. Thereafter events moved with almost suspicious speed, no doubt reflecting public outrage at the incident. On Thursday Bellingham's lawyers were told that they had been appointed by the court. The next day the trial began, a motion for postponement to allow time to bring certain defense witnesses to London having been denied.

At the trial a surgeon described Perceval's injuries in some detail and various witnesses told of the events surrounding the shooting. The prisoner spoke at length in his own behalf. Significantly, there was no expert testimony as to Bellingham's mental state. In his charge to the jury, Justice Mansfield stated: "The single question is, whether at the time this fact was committed, he [Bellingham] possessed a sufficient degree of understanding to distinguish good from evil, right from wrong, and whether murder was a crime not only against the law of God but against the law of this country." The jury found him guilty. Sentenced to death, Bellingham went to the gallows on Monday, 18 May (*OB,* May 1812: pp. 263–74; Quen, 1974).

In a subsequent case, psychiatric testimony brought acquittal. Thomas Rhodes escaped from St. Luke's Hospital for Lunatics and

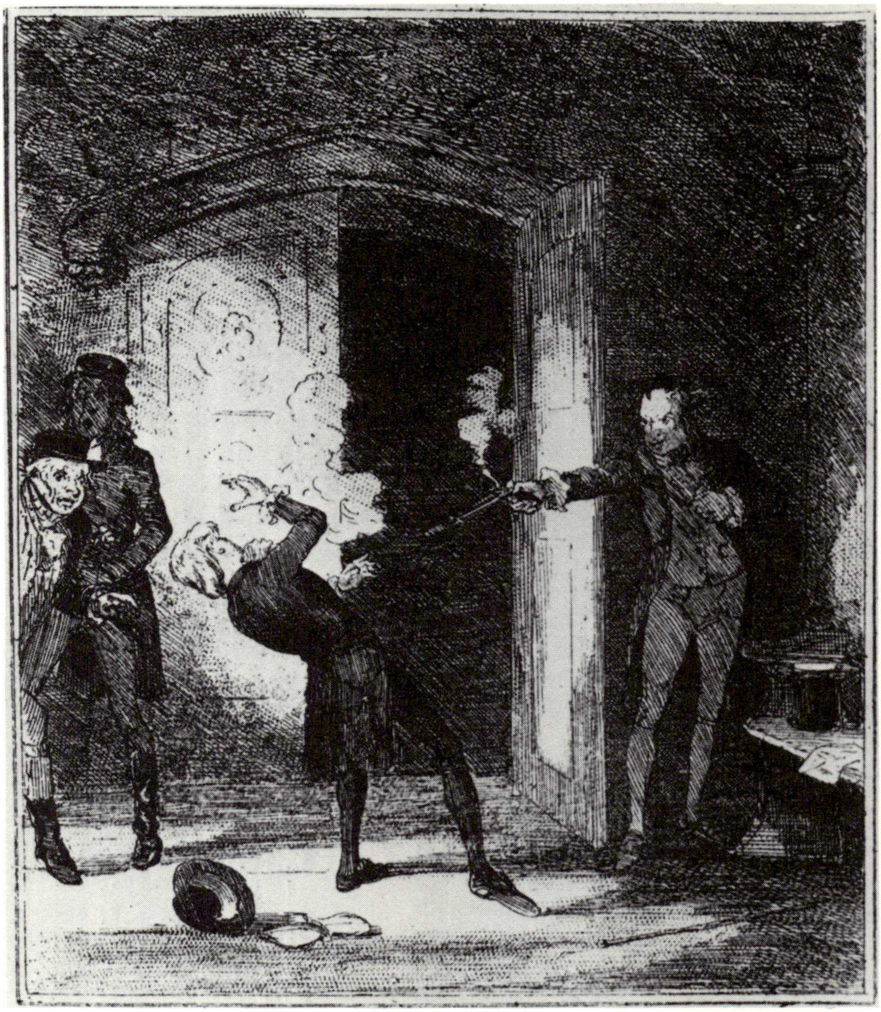

The Assassination of Perceval

subsequently shot and killed a man. At Rhodes's trial for murder, Dr. Sutherland, physician to St. Luke's, said Rhodes "has been under my care during the time he has been confined there. I saw him every Monday, and in my judgment he was insane the whole of the time. I should consider it imprudent that he should be at large. He certainly was not capable of judging whether his actions were right or wrong."

Two other experts who testified were William Nevly and John

Haslam, apothecaries at St. Luke's and Bethlehem Hospitals, respectively. They entirely agreed with Sutherland. Haslam described the prisoner as an incurable lunatic: "on my certificate he was put into Hoxton mad-house." Rhodes was found not guilty on the ground of insanity (*OB,* Dec. 1813: pp. 9–15).

John Haslam (1764–1844) after medical training had served for many years as apothecary to Bethlehem Hospital. In 1816 he received an honorary M.D. degree from the University of Aberdeen. Thereupon he set up practice as a physician in London, utilizing his extensive practical experience in the care of the insane, and in 1817 published *Medical Jurisprudence as It Relates to Insanity.* He had definite views regarding the testimony of the psychiatrist:

> When a medical person is employed concerning any one to whom insanity is imputed, his principal enquiry is concerning his insanity; it is not his object to ascertain how much reason he possesses, but how far, and on what topic he is insane. And having gauged his insanity, he has performed his duty. If it should be presumed that any medical practitioner is able to penetrate into the recesses of a lunatic's mind . . . and to depose that he knew the *Good* and *Evil, Right* and *Wrong,* he was about to commit, it must be confessed that such knowledge is beyond the limits of our attainment. (Haslam, in Cooper, 1819: p. 294)

A member of the nobility was again the target of a would-be assassin on 8 April 1818 when David Davis fired a badly loaded pistol at Lord Palmerston (1784–1865), Secretary of War and later Prime Minister, at the War Office. Davis, seized immediately, was tried the following month for attempted murder. Astley Cooper, one of London's leading surgeons, testified that His Lordship's injury was a bruise caused by a ball from a pistol. A police officer who had searched the prisoner's lodgings told of finding a pistol with powder and bullets, as well as various papers including, curiously enough, *The Trial of Bellingham.* It developed that Davis had been a lieutenant in the 62nd Regiment and had been "returned," that is, reported, to Palmerston as insane, early in 1816.

Davis's defense at his trial was not entirely coherent. He alleged that he could prove his insanity, that he had a grievance against Palmerston, and that he had suffered greatly. The report in the *Sessions Papers* indicates that upon the evidence of a surgeon, a clergyman, and five laymen, all of whom believed Davis to be a lunatic, he was found not guilty "*on the ground that they* [the members of the jury] *believed him to be insane at the time he committed the act*" (*OB,* May 1818: pp. 250–52).

PHYSICAL CAUSATION OF INSANITY

Unusually brutal homicides allegedly committed by female lunatics were ascribed by medical witnesses to the heredity of the accused and to lactational insanity or puerperal mania (*OB*, May 1822: pp. 330–31; Jan. 1835: pp. 410–14) or to mania resulting from suppression of menstruation due to conception or menopause (*OB*, July 1862: pp. 300–13). Insanity in a male was attributed to *recovery* from dysentery—"its being attended with bleeding would be very beneficial to his state of mind; it would improve it; and on his getting stronger, the delusion would be more likely to return" (*OB*, Sept. 1827: pp. 625–28). Some forms of lunacy were thus believed to have a physical basis (R. Smith, 1981: p. 40). At the same time physicians were struggling to classify mental disease, using a taxonomic scheme something like that employed in botany. Mental conditions were categorized on the basis of symptoms rather than etiology. William Cullen, a leader in the movement, "rejected the psychological causation of some disorders and favored a cerebral aetiology" (Howells and Osborn, 1975: p. 190). G. E. Male stated that the two chief kinds of insanity were mania and melancholia, to which might be added dementia or fatuity, that is, imbecility (1819: p. 247).

MORAL INSANITY

In 1835 a mental disease termed "moral insanity" was described by James Cowles Prichard (1786–1848). This remarkable Bristol physician, philogist, and ethnologist published his *Treatise on Insanity and Other Disorders Affecting the Mind* in 1835 only after years of experience with lunatic patients.

Prichard distinguished between intellectual insanity and insanity of the emotions and will (Tuke, 1909: 16, 344–46; R. Smith, 1981: pp. 38–40). Intellectual insanity, in turn, was divided into monomania (an illness dominated by one idea or subject), mania, and dementia. In addition there was moral insanity, which in D. H. Tuke's words, was "not necessarily the concomitant or outcome of mental disorder or incapacity." The concept of moral insanity seems to have represented recognition of the failure of moral judgment without such concurrent "amount of intellectual disorder as would be legally recognised either in a court of law or for the purpose of certification" (p. 345). In 1842 Prichard discussed the medicolegal aspects of moral insanity in a book, *On the Different Forms of Insanity, in Relation to Jurisprudence*. The concept of moral insanity was to be debated for decades to come.

EDWARD OXFORD

On 10 June 1840 Edward Oxford, a half-caste potboy aged eighteen or nineteen, fired two pistols at Queen Victoria in her carriage. There was afterward some question as to whether the pistols were loaded with bullets. In any event, neither Victoria nor anyone else was injured. Oxford freely admitted his act. Having been indicted for treason, he was allowed to have counsel. Rallied for the defense at his trial were numerous relatives and friends and four distinguished physicians. The events of the shooting were established, and a police inspector testified that in Oxford's room assorted weapons and ammunition had been found, together with papers listing the rules, regulations, and officers (with fictitious names) of "Young England," apparently a secret military organization of which Oxford dreamed. The prisoner's mother told of his bizarre actions and suicide threats.

The medical experts who testified, although agreeing to Oxford's insanity, offered diverse reasons for their conclusions. Indeed their various theories comprised a fair sampling of contemporary psychiatric thought. Dr. John Birt Davis, a physician, was asked whether, if he saw a person fire a loaded pistol at the Queen in her carriage and

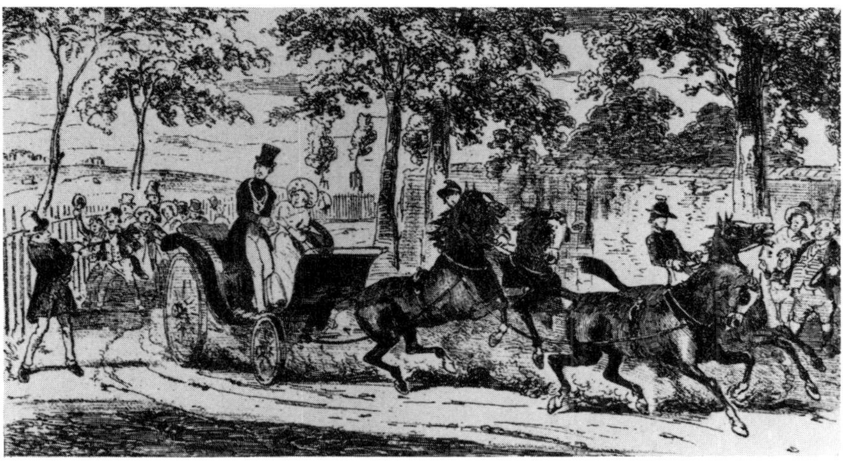

Oxford Shooting at the Queen

afterward "remain on the spot, [he would] declare he was the person who did it—to take pains to have that known . . . . would you refer such conduct to a sound or unsound state of mind? . . . *A*. I should judge him to be insane upon those facts alone." The distinguished pathologist Thomas Hodgkin (1798–1866), also appearing as a witness, was unknown as a specialist in mental disease. Nonetheless, Hodgkin implied that he considered the prisoner to be unbalanced—"I think that committing a crime without any apparent motive is an indication of insanity"—and offered learned remarks on what he termed "lesion of the will" (Allderidge, 1974).

Dr. John Conolly, a well-known Victorian physician and psychiatrist who had much to do with introducing humane treatment of the mentally ill, was physician to the Hanwell Lunatic Asylum. He had interviewed Oxford two days before the trial. Conolly considered him insane, adding a phrenological evaluation: "I examined the prisoner's head—it appeared to me that the formation of the anterior part of the head would indicate an imperfect development of a certain portion of the brain—I frequently find that form of head in insane persons—there are many persons of that form of head who are not insane."

Dr. Chowne, physican and lecturer on medical jurisprudence at Charing Cross Hospital, testified that he considered Oxford's state of mind "essentially unsound; there seems a mixture of insanity with imbecility." He referred to Oxford's type of lunacy as "*lesion* of the will . . . it has been called moral insanity."

Eventually the jury found the prisoner not guilty by reason of insanity. He was confined at Bethlehem Hospital, where Hadfield was also an inmate, until 1864, when the criminal patients at that place were moved to Broadmoor. By this time Oxford had learned six foreign languages, was accomplished at fives, chess, and draughts as well as at carpentry, house painting, and knitting, and was studying the violin.[9]

THE M'NAUGHTEN CASE

Medicolegal concepts of insanity and the insanity defense were to be greatly influenced by the trial in 1843 of Daniel M'Naughten[10] and its

9. *OB*, July 1840: pp. 465–510; Biggs, 1955: pp. 94–95; Jones, 1955: pp. 207–09; Allderidge, 1974.

10. Also spelled M'Naghten, McNaughton, etc.

sequelae.[11] The Scottish wood turner, aged twenty-seven, suffered from paranoid schizophrenia. One of his delusions was of persecution by the Tories. He came to London, and on 20 January 1843 shot Edward Drummond, Private Secretary to Robert Peel, then Prime Minister, apparently under the impression that Drummond was Peel. M'Naughten, who made his assault only a few feet away from a police constable, was at once arrested. Drummond died five days later.

M'Naughten's trial for murder began on 3 March at the Old Bailey. Although counsel was not assigned by the court, the prisoner was well represented by legal advisors, probably at the instigation of his father, since the accused man was not capable of acting on his own behalf. When the proceedings began, the police and other witnesses established the circumstances of the attack, about which there was little disagreement. Bransby Cooper, nephew of Sir Astley Cooper, told of extracting the pistol ball from the wound and of the sensible forensic precaution he thereupon took—"I believe this to be the mark I made on it [the ball] the day following." Nothing was said of autopsy findings except that the ball had penetrated the trunk from back to front, wounding the diaphragm.

Lay witnesses for the defense, including the father and several acquaintances of the accused, the Lord Provost of Glasgow, and the Commissioner of Police for Glasgow, all testified to M'Naughten's abnormal behavior. Alexander Cockburn, chief counsel for the defense, quoted at some length from Isaac Ray's *Medical Jurisprudence of Insanity* (1838).

Five medical men had interviewed M'Naughten in prison before the trial, Edward Thomas Monro,[12] Sir Alexander Morrison, M.D., and Mr. William M'Clewer for the defense and Doctors Bright and Sutherland for the prosecution. Monro represented the fifth generation of his family to specialize in the care of lunatics and to serve as physician to Bethlehem Hospital. On another occasion during his confinement M'Naughten had been examined by William Hutchinson, M.D., physician to the Royal Lunatic Asylum at Glasgow, John Crawford, Lecturer on Medical Jurisprudence at the Andersonian University of Glasgow, and Gilbert M'Murdo, surgeon of Newgate. All these experts except Bright and Sutherland testified, and all agreed that M'Naughten was insane.

11. Biggs, 1955: pp. 95–115; Jones, 1955: pp. 209–13; Dreher, 1967; Quen, 1968, 1974; Lewinstein, 1969: pp. 280–83; Allderidge, 1974; Simpson, 1975: pp. 239–41; Ficarra, 1977: pp. 5–16; Ormrod, 1977: pp. 6–11; R. Smith, 1981: p. 76.

12. Misspelled as "Monroe" in the *Sessions Papers*.

Aston Key, a surgeon at Guy's Hospital, and Forbes Winslow, physician and author of *The Plea of Insanity in Criminal Cases* (1843), had not examined the prisoner but did attend the trial. When called to the witness box, they concurred in the opinion of their colleagues as to M'Naughten's mental state.

The expert medical testimony was necessarily lengthy. Monro seemed to base his diagnosis of the prisoner largely on the repeated indications of paranoia:

> *Q*. Do you believe, judging from all the evidence, and your own investigation and inquiry of his state of mind, that the delusion in his mind operated to the extent of depriving him of all self-control? *A*. I do—it was the crowning act of his delusion—it was the climax of the whole matter, the carrying out of that precise idea which had been haunting him for years.
>
> *Q*. Is it now an established principle in the pathology of insanity that there may exist a partial delusion sufficient to overcome a man's moral sense and self-control, and render him irresponsible for his actions, exciting a partial insanity only, although the rest of the faculties of the mind may remain in all their ordinary state of operation? *A*. Yes, it is quite recognised—the distinction between monomania and general mania is quite recognised.

After hearing the massive testimony from the defense, Lord Chief Justice Tindal learned from the Solicitor General that he had no evidence or witnesses to refute it. The Chief Justice thereupon interrupted the trial and charged the jury. At his direction the members brought in a verdict of "not guilty, being insane" (*OB,* Feb. 1843: pp. 721–63). M'Naughten spent his remaining years in confinement, first at Bethlehem Hospital and then at Broadmoor.

The trial of course had attracted much attention, and the verdict quickly aroused an atmosphere of deep public concern, almost of panic. There was a general feeling, encouraged by the press, that M'Naughten should have been "punished"—permanent detainment in an asylum was not enough. Even the queen was moved to send a letter of protest to Sir Robert Peel, her Prime Minister. Although the opinion of the experts as to M'Naughten's insanity had been unanimous and strong, the decision of the judge to interrupt the trial before the medical issues had been fully explored was resented. After all, neither the prisoner's ability to distinguish right from wrong nor the issues of partial insanity and monomania had been properly debated, and two medical witnesses for the prosecution had not even been heard. There was anger that Key and Winslow, the two medical men who had observed the prisoner in court but had never previously seen him, had been allowed to testify.

On 6 March 1843, three days after the trial began, the issue was raised in the House of Lords. As a result, the fifteen judges of the Queen's Bench were assembled by the Lord Chancellor and met in an effort, in effect, to define the law of insanity. Eleven of the judges were able to agree on four principles, later to be known as the "M'Naughten rules." The eleven declared that "the jury ought to be told in all cases that every man is presumed to be sane, and to possess a sufficient degree of reason to be responsible for his crimes, until the contrary be proved to their satisfaction." The learned judges continued: "to establish a defence on the ground of insanity, it must be clearly proved, that, at the time of the committing of the act, the party accused was labouring under such a defect of reason, from disease of the mind, as not to know the nature and quality of the act he was doing, or, if he did know it, that he did not know he was doing what was wrong." If a person who committed an offense suffered from a

> partial delusion only, and is not in other respects insane, we think he must be considered in the same situation as to responsibility as if the facts with respect to which the delusion exists were real. For example, if under the influence of his delusion, he supposes another man to be in the act of attempting to take away his life, and he kills that man, as he supposes, in self-defence, he would be exempt from punishment. If his delusion was that the deceased had inflicted a serious injury to his character and fortune, and he killed him in revenge for such supposed injury, he would be liable to punishment.

Finally, the judges responded to the question:

> Can a medical man, conversant with the disease of insanity, who never saw the prisoner previously to the trial, but was present during the whole trial and the examination of all the witnesses, be asked his opinion as to the state of the prisoner's mind at the time of the commission of the alleged crime, or his opinion whether the prisoner was conscious at the time of doing the act that he was acting contrary to law, or whether he was labouring under any and what delusion at the time?

The answer was that, yes, the medical man could give his opinion on these matters, but only if "the facts are admitted, or not disputed, so that the question is purely a scientific one" (Wallis, 1892: 4, cols. 847–48, 931–32).

The influence of the M'Naughten rules continues to this day. Although they were and are criticized, it must be conceded that they represented a concerted effort to clarify a murky and troublesome situation. Historically, they should be seen against the background of the period, reflecting the prevalent concern with the threat to public safety imposed by any unrestrained and dangerous lunatic. As Quen has pointed out (1968):

> The temper of the time appeared to require the reassurance of definite and explicit rules. It was a time of violent ideas, violent feelings, and violent acts . . . . The anxiety about lawless violence found a target in the M'Naughten verdict. Like a lens, it focused attention on the violent and criminally insane, and on what protection the law offered society. That protection was seen as directly proportional to the stringency of the law.

As the courts struggled to define legal insanity, so did medicine continue to strive to understand, categorize, and diagnose mental diseases. For example, the concept of the compartmentalized mind was further examined. It was believed, as it may still be, that some areas of an individual's mind could be sane while other parts were insane (Biggs, 1955: p. 72). "The criminal may be mad on one subject only, and that may be the subject of his crime" (Conolly, 1830: p. 451). Because it was thought that such insanity was compartmentalized, it followed that monomania might go entirely unsuspected until suddenly it burst forth (Foucault, 1978). Homicidal monomania, said Alfred Swaine Taylor, much respected for his grasp of criminal insanity, could appear at any age, even in young children (1856: p. 655).

One result of the inability of the medical profession to agree on the diagnosis of insanity was that careful medical evaluation of an accused person occasionally was neither attempted nor requested. The implication was that sensible laymen could do as well as the doctors. Consider an example. A forty-five-year-old man beat a thirteen-year-old girl to death with exceptional savagery. He was indicted for intent to murder, to disable, and to do some grievous bodily harm. It developed that he had been confined for eight months in a private lunatic asylum. It was further deposed that he suffered from uncontrolled fits of rage and that after he was arrested for injuring the child, "he said it was not he that did it, it was God did it, and that fire came down from heaven that morning—he said that the Royal family were all dead, Prince Albert and all."

The only medical opinion came from a surgeon who had attended the *victim* in the hospital but who had not even seen the assailant. This witness was asked, "Is causeless violence one of the symptoms of insanity? *A*. I should say so—I have had very little knowledge of cases of insanity—if he had no object in view in thus injuring the girl I should say it would indicate insanity." Then four long-time lay friends of the accused took their turns in the witness box. One admitted that the accused had fits of irrationality; the others asserted that they never knew him to be insane. The jury found the prisoner guilty only on the count of grievous bodily harm, and he received a sentence of twelve months in prison (*OB,* Nov. 1843: pp. 29–31). The trial affords interesting contrasts to that of M'Naughten, held only a few months earlier.

Strange medical theories continued to be heard. A woman suffered a severe head injury. Some months later she cut her own throat and those of her two children with a razor. The children died, but the mother recovered. Subsequently her mind allegedly cleared—"she certainly seemed better." Her fit of insanity was ascribed by a physician to brain fever. He was asked on the stand:

> Have you had considerable experience, and paid attention to cases of persons affected with insanity?—*A.* Yes, and have had insane persons under my charge in my house—insanity exhibits itself in a variety of forms; sometimes in the form of constitutional imbecility; sometimes from local causes; sometimes from disorganization of the brain . . . . a person labouring under insanity arising from pressure of blood on the brain would be relieved extensively and speedily by liberal blood-letting—a person in that state cutting her own throat would be very much relieved.

The prisoner was found not guilty by reason of insanity (*OB,* Mar. 1884: pp. 724–30).

ROBERT PATE

An alternative to not seeking an expert medical opinion was to ignore it. On 27 June 1850 Queen Victoria, riding in her carriage, was struck on the head with a small cane by one Robert Pate. The assailant, aged thirty, was at once arrested by a policeman named James Silver, the same individual, it developed, who had seized M'Naughten more than seven years earlier after he had shot Edward Drummond. The right side of the queen's forehead was cut and bruised, but not seriously. Apparently her horsehair bonnet, supported by a wire frame, had absorbed some of the force of the blow.

It came out at his trial that Pate had been an officer in the 10th Hussars from 1841 to 1846. At first he had discharged his duties satisfactorily, but later became increasingly depressed and resentful. He complained that he was being poisoned, that "his stomach and bowels were full of bricks, and that the doctor had not the skill to remove them." In 1845 he left the regiment. Instances of bizarre actions continued.

One of the medical men who testified at Pate's trial was John Conolly, M.D. He had seen the accused three times since his arrest. In Conolly's opinion, Pate knew the difference between right and wrong, did not when interviewed suffer from delusion, and recognized that he had done wrong in attacking the queen, although he could not explain his act. Edward T. Monro, M.D., who had had five meetings in prison with the prisoner, in general agreed with Conolly, adding "I think that a man conceiving he had bricks and stones in his stomach, and being hunted by persons, and imagining that the cook and messman had conspired to poison him, are indications of insanity."

The judge at Pate's trial, Baron Alderson, had earlier made clear his disagreement with the verdict in the M'Naughten case, commenting from the bench, "I am aware of that decision, and am quite sure it was wrong, and the sooner it is corrected the better" (*OB,* Nov. 1849: p. 49).[13] Alderson again expressed his dissatisfaction with the medical interpretation of insanity when charging the jury during Pate's trial:

> The learned judge . . . observed . . . that it was not because a man was insane that he was unpunishable; and he must say that upon this point there was generally a very grievous delusion in the minds of medical men. "The only insanity which excused a man for his acts was that species of delusion which conduced and drove him to commit the act alleged against him. They ought to have a proof of a formed disease of the mind, a *disease existing before the act was committed,* and which made the person accused incapable of knowing at the time he did the act that it was a wrong act for him to do." (Taylor, 1856: p. 665)

Pate was found guilty and was sentenced to transportation for seven years (*OB,* July 1850: pp. 374–88).

RIGHT AND WRONG

The ability to distinguish between right and wrong was a crucial issue in 1851 in a complex arson case involving an occupied dwelling house. Testimony by firemen, a policeman, insurance company representa-

13. For a discussion of this and related juridical dissent see R. Smith, 1981: pp. 68, 78.

tives, a surveyor, and other revealed many details of how the fire was set, turpentine being the principal incendiary agent. James Huggins, the accused, was clearly paranoid. At his trial four physicians in succession stepped to the witness stand to describe his mental state at various times during the preceding two years as suicidal, excited, depressed, and confused. However, John Conolly and also Sir Alexander Morrison, M.D., physician to Bethlehem Hospital and probably the best qualified of the four, repeatedly evaded efforts of the prosecution to extract an unqualified statement as to whether Huggins could distinguish right from wrong. Morrison, hard pressed, gave voice to the doctor's dilemma: "I am not here to decide the question of responsibility in an insane person, and therefore I cannot go to the length of answering what lawyers frequently ask, is he capable of distinguishing between right and wrong; I mean to say his brain is in a disordered state, but I cannot define the degree of responsibility and consciousness which he possesses." The third medical witness had not seen the prisoner for three years and wisely declined to say whether the accused knew right from wrong at the time he was arrested. The fourth expert reluctantly conceded that the prisoner did know the difference, "as do a great many decided lunatics." Huggins was sentenced to death (*OB,* July 1851: pp. 355–72).

In this and other cases of the period, although the doctors strove to limit their testimony to describing symptoms which supported a *medical* diagnosis of insanity, in court the *legal* criterion was the ability to distinguish right from wrong. The influence of the M'Naughten rules continued.

PRISON SURGEONS

Walker calls attention to the emergence of the prison surgeon as a forensic psychiatric witness (1968: p. 84). This official could, apparently at his discretion, interview prisoners during the pretrial period of their incarceration. Gilbert Wakefield MacMurdo (1799–1869), for some years surgeon to Newgate Gaol, as early as 1830 was occasionally giving expert testimony at the Old Bailey (*OB,* Dec. 1830: pp. 88–91) and continued to do so until 1843 or later (*OB,* Feb. 1843: pp. 721–63). Apparently his position at the prison was not full-time, as he accepted an appointment as assistant surgeon at St. Thomas's Hospital in 1841 (Power, 1930: *2,* 110).

John Rowland Gibson (1814–92) became a surgeon at Newgate in

1854 (*OB*, Aug. 1872: p. 314) and seems to have served there for the rest of his life (Power, 1930: *1* p. 441). He also on many occasions was an expert witness regarding the mental state of prisoners, appearing in this capacity as early as 1856 (*OB*, Jan. 1856: pp. 296–302).

REGISTRATION AND LICENSURE

The history of the management of public and private mental asylums is beyond the scope of this book, but it is of interest that forensic medical testimony was given at the trial of Sophia Leander at the Old Bailey for "Unlawfully receiving at the same time two or more lunatics into her house, it not being registered or licensed for that purpose." Dr. Thomas Christie, resident medical superintendent of Penley House, Hackney, an institution caring for 140 to 150 lunatics, made an inspection of Sion House, Mrs. Leander's establishment, in April 1864 in company with one of the Commissioners in Lunacy. Sion House accommodated about eighty patients; Christie interviewed a number of them. Judging from his testimony, he was not concerned with the physical conditions of the establishment but rather with the mental state of the patients, which ranged from delusional to imbecile. Mrs. Leander was found guilty and was placed in penalty of a judgment if her house was not closed (*OB*, June 1864: pp. 116–18).

A few months later Henry Wilkins was indicted for providing board and lodging for a deranged woman. The problem was that she was not certified as a lunatic and that Wilkins's house was not licensed for the care of the insane. Two surgeons and three physicians testified that the woman was indeed "of unsound mind and not able to take care of herself." Wilkins was found guilty, but judgment was deferred (*OB*, Sept. 1864: pp. 402–09). In a similar trial a few years after this, Thomas Harrington Tuke, M.D.,[14] son-in-law of John Conolly, testified to the imbecility of a woman who was said to be unlawfully lodged in the house of one John H. Harris (*OB*, Feb. 1867: pp. 486–92). In this case the defendant escaped on a legal technicality.

THE INSANITY DEFENSE IN LATER YEARS

The insanity defense was undertaken occasionally in assault and homicide trials in later decades, usually with success. An exception was the

14. Tuke (1826–88), son of Edward Francis Tuke, came of Irish parents and was not related to Daniel Hack Tuke and other members of the Yorkshire family that did so much to improve the care of the insane in England (Hunter and Macalpine, 1961).

case of John Selby Watson, tried at the Old Bailey in 1872 for the murder of Anne Watson, his wife, by multiple blows to the head. He left a note that he had killed her "in a fit of rage to which she provoked me," and then attempted to commit suicide by ingesting prussic acid. Watson, a sixty-seven-year-old schoolmaster, had been depressed following his discharge from his teaching position. At the trial Dr. George P. Rugg, a general practitioner, claimed that the prisoner suffered from melancholia, homicidal mania, and suicidal mania. However, experts appearing for the prosecution, Edmund Pope, a police surgeon, Dr. Thomas H. Waterworth, surgeon at Horsemonger Lane Gaol, where the prisoner was confined, Dr. Edgar Shepherd, medical superintendent at the Hanwell Lunatic Asylum, and John Rowland Gibson, surgeon of Newgate, agreed that Watson's mind was sound. Then Dr. Henry Maudsley,[15] Dr. George F. Blandford, and Dr. Joseph Rogers, all experienced alienists, agreed that Watson suffered from melancholia and was of unsound mind. One can readily picture the dilemma of the jury of laymen, obliged to make a choice between the opposed and highly technical opinions of the experts. The jurymen found Watson guilty, and he was sentenced to death (*OB*, Jan. 1872: pp. 147–90).

The hereditary nature of insanity continued to be an issue when the defense could point to mentally disturbed relatives of the accused person. Said the brother of a prisoner, for example, "my mother died of an epileptic fit . . . . I have had one fit myself, about seven years back—my uncle William died in Bethlehem . . . before that he had been confined in Guy's Hospital under restraint, in a straight waistcoat and fastened down to the bedstead." Dr. Thomas H. Tuke testified that he would consider as an important element "in this or any case a very strong hereditary tendency to insanity, and epilepsy and insanity are most frequent concomitants of homicidal mania—epileptic mania is a most dangerous malady in references to the lives of others and themselves, and it is frequently hereditary" (*OB*, Dec. 1874: pp. 150–67).

THE O'DONNELL TRIAL

The later operation of the M'Naughten rules is well illustrated by the trial in 1876 of Charles O'Donnell, aged fifty-seven, for the murder of

15. A leader in contemporary psychiatric thought, Maudsley (1835–1918) was much interested in medicolegal problems. He was the founder of the psychiatric hospital which bears his name.

his wife. On Thursday, 26 October, the couple were heard to quarrel in their lodgings. Mrs. O'Donnell was not seen alive again after that day. On Sunday, the twenty-ninth, the husband, somewhat intoxicated, had tea with his neighbor. Asked about Mrs. O'Donnell, the husband responded, "I hope she is in heaven by this." The next morning her partly decomposed body was found in the room, completely disordered, where the O'Donnells had lodged. Several skull fractures, apparently inflicted with a poker, were discovered. It was estimated by a physician that death had occurred at least three days earlier. The husband, again intoxicated, was arrested and charged with murder.

At the trial a surgeon named Dover, a self-described specialist for almost twenty years in the treatment of insanity, and William Smiles, surgeon to the Middlesex House of Correction, indicated that they had seen the prisoner several times in the preceding months. They were aware that he had suffered from sunstroke in India. Smiles remembered O'Donnell as

> a man of sound mind and understanding, he always talked quite collectedly and showed no symptoms of insanity whatever . . . . I have a great deal of practice in cases of insanity . . . . I know that he attempted to commit suicide, and that he has been in Colney Hatch [Lunatic Asylum] for three months—I have frequently known cases where a man has been in a Lunatic Asylum, and has left cured, and the mania has broken out again—in a man who has suffered from sunstroke in India, and afterwards become insane, and who has been confined, the fit of insanity would no doubt be likely to recur again.

Dover agreed with this opinion.

John Roland Gibson, surgeon of Newgate, had visited O'Donnell daily from 9 November, when he was committed to that prison, to 23 November, when the trial began; "during that time I saw nothing to lead me to the belief that he was anything but a man of sound mind and understanding . . . . in a man who has suffered from sunstroke, and who has been insane, madness may very likely be brought on again, in my opinion, by drinking and excitement, it would be very likely to bring it on."

Frederick Thomas Coates, another surgeon, had treated O'Donnell on 8 May 1875 for a deep incised wound of the forearm. "I had some conversation with him about it; he said that he wished to die, and he wanted to go to heaven, and that some spirit came down and told him to do it."

The jury soon agreed that O'Donnell was guilty of murder. However, after deliberating for an hour, the jurymen were forced to send a letter to the presiding judge, Mr. Baron Hawkins. The response reveals the court's interpretation of the M'Naughten rules:

> Gentlemen, I have had a communication from you, and I understand your question to be this, that having no evidence of the actual state of mind of the prisoner *at the time he committed the act* [italics added], you wish to know whether you may entertain a presumption of insanity; it is my duty to tell you, that the law presumes that every man is responsible for his actions, and if you have no evidence at all as to the state of mind of the prisoner at the time he caused this catastrophe, you are bound to say he is guilty, if you believe that he caused the act of death. A man who wants to shift from himself the responsibility he incurs by causing the death of another, is bound by affirmative evidence to satisfy the Jury that, at the time he committed the act, he did not know the character of the act he was doing, and did not know he was doing a wrong act; it is for him to prove it, and if he fails to prove it to your satisfaction, you have no alternative but to find him guilty of the offence; that is the law on the subject.

The jury accordingly returned a verdict of guilty, and O'Donnell was sentenced to death (*OB,* Nov. 1876: pp. 37–45). No one could prove that he was not sane at the time of the murder.

The foregoing pages survey forensic medicine in relation to insanity, by no means comprehensively, up to 1878. We have seen that by the fourteenth century, lunacy had been accepted in law as a reason for not punishing an offender. Thereafter the duty of the court was clear enough in the trial of demonstrably unbalanced persons charged with a felony. Problems arose, however, in the case of accused persons who were by legal standards perhaps insane, or *sometimes* insane, and whose conduct most of the time fell within the wide range generally regarded as normal. For, as John Rowland Gibson conceded, the "boundaries between sanity and insanity are very ill defined." An accused person perceived to stand on one side of a changeable and imprecise line was held not responsible for his actions; on the other side he was in peril of his life. It was at this interface that law and medicine met, the one to define the boundary, the other to determine if it had been crossed. In practice, the two disciplines were driven to try reluctantly to solve together the problem that confronted both.

From the medical standpoint, the chief difficulty was the accurate *diagnosis* of insanity in all its forms. Mental disease was poorly understood, and some symptoms were ill defined and arguable. It is not surprising that reputable, experienced, and, for their day, competent alienists found themselves contradicting each other in court. Unlike the tangible signs of a shooting or stabbing or strangling, few of the symptoms of madness could be measured or be revealed by post-mortem examination or even be described in precise terms.

Looking back, we are reminded also that until the latter part of the eighteenth century it was unusual for a *medical* judgment as to the state of mind of a prisoner even to be heard in court. By the lay mind and often by the judicial mind, insanity was seldom regarded as a medical matter. Lunatics who fell afoul of the law were generally confined with other offenders in prison and received no special attention except for harsh restraints for the violent and uncooperative. Insanity might be a social and legal problem, but it was seldom seen as a medical one. This helps to explain why on occasion a judge, after hearing the testimony only of laymen, would take it on himself to rule as to the sanity of a prisoner at the bar. When, finally, expert medical opinion began to be sought in lunacy cases, the physician or surgeon would venture a judgment only as to *whether* the accused was sane. Not until the nineteenth century did medical witnesses begin to explain *why* they had reached their conclusions.

Meanwhile, by necessity, the law was applying its own tests of insanity. Their enumeration by Lodge (1901) may be summarized as follows:

> The "boy of fourteen" test, derived from Sir Matthew Hale's seventeenth-century inquiry as to whether a person "labouring under melancholy distempers, hath yet ordinarily as great understanding as a child of fourteen years."
>
> The "wild beast" test, originating in Justice Tracey's charge to the jury at the trial of Edwin Arnold in 1724: Does the culprit "know what he is doing any more than an infant, a brute, or a wild beast"?
>
> The "sane mind at the time of the act" test: Lord Chief Justice Kenyon at the trial of Hadfield in 1800 related the culpability of the accused to "whether, at the very time when he committed the act, his mind was sane."
>
> The "right or wrong" test: At the trial of Bellingham in 1812, Sir James Mansfield raised a question as to whether the prisoner knew in principle the difference between right and wrong.
>
> The "sane intellect" test, growing out of the M'Naughten trial in 1843, asked whether the allegedly insane person knew "the nature and quality of his act." This criterion continued to be applied for about fifty years.

Clearly the jurists struggled on a path no less uncertain than that of their medical colleagues.

X

Other Forensic Medical Problems

NONFATAL ASSAULTS

In law, the threat to use force to injure another person is *assault*; the attack itself is *battery*. In this book the term *assault* is used in the popular sense to represent the physical attack. Fatal assaults of course were prosecuted as homicides. Nonfatal assaults with injury that ended in trials at the Old Bailey were numerous (table 9) and often shared common characteristics. One or more of the persons involved was intoxicated. The attacks were committed on impulse and in anger. The weapon was an object conveniently at hand. The proclivity of males for violence was much greater than that of females (table 10).

Trials for nonfatal assaults on children were relatively uncommon, for which several reasons come to mind. Infants and children were less able than adults to defend themselves, and attacks on the young were more likely to result in homicide. In addition, testimony repeatedly indicated that attackers attempted to conceal violence directed toward children, which in turn suggests that in other assaults on children efforts to conceal violence and its results may well have been successful. If so, the actual *incidence* of nonfatal attacks on children was higher than prosecutions in court would indicate.

Injuries inflicted in attacks on adults were most often to the head, especially the top of the head, the face, and the anterior neck, and to the hands, which were traumatized when the victim tried to protect himself or herself from a weapon. Nonfatal assaults with a knife or blunt object were similar to those described in chapter 2 (assaults with

Table 9. Old Bailey Trials for Assault with Nonfatal Injury, 1729–1878

	Medical testimony	No medical testimony	Total
1729–38		4	4
1739–48[a]		1	1
1749–58		6	6
1759–68	1	6	7
1769–78	1	2	3
1779–88		1	1
1789–98	1		1
1799–08	4	4	8
1809–18	8	13	21
1819–28	15	18	33
1829–38	42	53	95
1839–48	279	71	350
1849–58	267	46	313
1859–68	273	44	317
1869–78	188	47	235
Total	1079	316	1395

[a]Incomplete; some *Sessions Papers* missing.

firearms will be discussed later in this chapter). Wounds occasionally became grossly infected (see below). The victim of an assault could usually describe the attacker and some of the circumstances. Expert medical witnesses were likely to speak of nonfatal injuries in less detail than would have been usual for a homicide. Indeed, during much of the eighteenth century medical testimony often was not elicited in assault cases. Such evidence was first given at the Old Bailey in 1765,

Table 10. Sex of Attackers and Victims in Assaults with Nonfatal Injury, Old Bailey, 1809–41

	Assaults
Male(s) attacked male(s)	63
Male(s) attacked female(s)	22
Female(s) attacked male(s)	11
Female(s) attacked female(s)	8
Male and female attacked male	2
Total	110

and did not become common until the second decade of the nineteenth century (table 9).

Assaults with corrosive substances, unlike most attacks, were usually premeditated. Eight attacks made with acid or ammonia came to trial. For example, a servant girl who, judging from the testimony, may well have been insane, poured "sulphuric acid" into the mouth of a five-week-old baby. Medical examination showed acid burns of the skin of the cheek and mucosa of the mouth. It is of interest that the acid was identified only by hearsay and by the surgeon cautiously tasting it (*OB*, Jan. 1853: pp. 296–301).

In other assaults, two men and a woman threw vitriol (sulfuric acid) at adult victims, causing burns of the face and neck. The attackers said that they used the acid in their work to clean bottles (*OB*, Sept. 1872: pp. 433–34), metal rails (*OB*, Sept. 1873: pp. 432–33), and tins (*OB*, Aug. 1877: pp. 300–03). In no case was the alleged sulfuric acid actually identified by chemical test. In an additional assault a man was temporarily blinded when a dilute solution of ammonia was thrown in his face (*OB*, Sept. 1873: pp. 449–56).

Christison described a case of a woman's premeditated attack with sulfuric acid in Edinburgh in 1827. A man's face was severely burned. About twelve hours after the assault he was bled from the arm for relief from pain. On the fifth day soreness and inflammation developed at the site of the phlebotomy. The infection progressed, and the patient succumbed on the thirteenth day, death being ascribed "to the inflammation of the arm and concomitant fever." This diagnosis was confirmed at autopsy. Chemical tests established the presence of sulfuric acid residue in burned, but not unburned, portions of the victim's hat and coat. Christison pointed out that this crime raised "a nice legal question, as to the responsibility of the prisoner for an event [the death from sepsis] which depended only indirectly on the injury inflicted by her, and directly on an insignificant surgical operation [phlebotomy]." The prisoner in this case was not charged under Scottish law with homicide (Christison, 1829c: pp. 229–36).

WOUND INFECTION

Wound infection was a not unusual complication of injury. The term *infection,* incidentally, does not appear in the Old Bailey testimony that was reviewed. It must be remembered that Pasteur's proof that disease may be due to a living organism was not developed until the

1860s and 1870s and that Koch demonstrated the relation of micro-organisms to wound infection and sepsis only in 1878. Before this time medical men spoke of *inflammation, mortification,* and *gangrene,* of *erysipelas* and *lock jaw.* Precise definitions by our standards of these terms as used before the promulgation of the germ theory of disease is difficult. According to the 1868 edition of *Dunglison's Medical Dictionary,* in *inflammation* "altered nutrition in a part is occasioned by some agency:—owing to which the blood flows into the capillary vessels in greater abundance than natural . . . whence result pain, redness, heat, tension, and swelling." *Mortification* is defined as the "loss of vitality in a part of the body. The incipient stage of mortification, when the disease is still recoverable, is called Gangrene." *Erysipelas,* said Dunglison, is a disease characterized by cutaneous inflammation, fever, tension, swelling and heat of the affected area, pain, redness, and, frequently, small vesicles. Numerous varieties of erysipelas were recognized.

When inflammation followed a homicidal attack, the court was frequently concerned to know whether death was due to the original trauma, to the subsequent infection, or to both. For example, a soldier struck in the forehead with a broadsword during a quarrel suffered a wound exposing the brain as well as several cuts on the arm and shoulder. He rapidly became ill and so violent that he had to be restrained, dying three days after being injured. The surgeon explained the sequelae as he understood them. "*Bailey.* The mortal wound I take to be on the forehead, where the brains were laid open. All wounds, from pain, occasion a fluxion, and from thence arises an inflammation, which sometimes is carried off by a digestion, or matter [pus] running; but the brain was inflamed, and I believe a mortification ensued, for on his arm there appeared a tendency to mortification" (*OB,* Feb. 1748: pp. 106–07). Here was wound sepsis as seen through eighteenth-century eyes. What we would call infection was *expected* to occur. As late as 1868 Dunglison spoke of "pus of a good quality—*laudable pus, Pus bonum* sev *laudabile* . . . . Normal pus" (p. 817).

Compound fractures were known often to be followed by fatal inflammation, as in the case of a man whose leg was broken in a fight. His surgeon

> examined it very minutely, and I told his friends it would be mortal . . . a compound dislocation of the ancle is generally a mortal accident . . . .
>
> The danger you apprehended was a mortification?—I apprehended that would come on in three or four days.

> Would no amputation prevent that?—I have seen them amputated, but I spoke to Mr. Lock concerning it, and he said he would not do anything, for he could not save his life . . . . An inflammation came on, and that was the cause of his death. (*OB,* Sept. 1787: pp. 1036–39)

Erysipelas, St. Anthony's fire, mentioned repeatedly in connection with infections secondary to injury, was little understood:

> I believe erysipelas occurs from atmospheric causes, and that it will not follow from any wound unless those atmospheric causes are prevailing, and the constitution of the patient is in a condition to absorb that poison, whatever it may be. (*OB,* Mar. 1850: p. 553)

> It sometimes arises quite independent of any blow, from the constitution being reduced to a state of debility, and from intemperance, exposure, or any previous indisposition—I do not recollect ever seeing erysipelas in a child without a scratch or injury of some kind. (*OB,* Oct. 1854: p. 1395)

> There are two theories about erysipelas; one, that it arises with wounds, and one without; but with wounds they are more liable to erysipelas. (*OB,* Feb. 1875: p. 282)

The earlier textbooks of forensic medicine do not seem to mention wound infection under its various designations, but Taylor (1856: p. 250) warns that if a wounded individual should acquire gangrene or erysipelas because he or she was transported to a hospital where one of these diseases "is diffusing itself by infectious propagation," and if the victim should acquire the disease and die, the accused person may be held responsible for the fatality.

INJURIES BY FIRE

A young woman perished in a fire in a house on Oxford Street in 1832. Jonathan Smithies, tobacconist and cabinet maker, lived in the building and had his shop there. At the inquest the testimony of several witnesses made it clear that he was guilty of arson, and he was indicted for the woman's murder. It was learned that on the premises he had stored not only beeswax and turpentine, used in finishing furniture, but also sacks of shavings and a small quantity of gunpowder. A fireman found in the basement a contrivance of shavings and gunpowder obviously intended to start a fire. The device had been ignited but had gone out before it was consumed. Another fireman found kindling laid for a fire but only partly burned. There was no mention of an autopsy of the victim's badly burned body. However, the injuries of Smithies, the arsonist, provided much evidence for the medical observer. The tobacconist had become trapped during the fire under a grating. He was rescued and taken to Middlesex Hospital. Here a surgeon found that the man's

> hands were very much burnt, and his face also—those on the hands appeared ordinary burns—those on the face appeared peculiar; they appeared to be blue—there was a case of burning from gunpowder in the hospital in November last, and from the observation I made of this case, there was a similarity in some respects . . . . each of the prisoner's knees were burnt; he wore trousers, which were not at all burnt about the knees . . . . he wore long stockings, and neither of the stockings had any burn about the knee . . . . gunpowder will generally leave grains or marks in the face for some time after . . . .
>
> *Q*. Is it at all extraordinary for a man, ascending up a staircase, to have his hands and face burnt? *A*. Not without his clothes being burnt—I did not see his coat; he had not got it on when he was brought.

Defense counsel was trying to establish that Smithies had been burned, not by exploding gunpowder, but only while attempting to escape from the blazing house. But it developed that the prisoner had managed after being injured to replace his burned stockings and trousers with garments supplied by a neighbor.

Then an expert witness testified for the defense:

> RALPH HARRIES. I am an apothecary . . . . I have been accustomed to treat patients under the effects of injuries occasioned by explosions of gunpowder, and have always found we could not get rid of the blueness; there is not the least appearance in the prisoner's features to warrant an opinion that he has been burnt by an explosion of gunpowder; I have resided in the neighborhood of mines, and had great experience of such injuries . . . .
>
> MR. ADOLPHUS [prosecuting]. *Q*. Might not a small quantity of gunpowder have discoloured the skin, and be washed off? *A*. I have never seen a case where the skin has been broken, but it has always remained; if the skin was not broken, I suppose it would come off . . . .
>
> MR. LONSDALE. When he came to the hospital, his face was discoloured; it was a grey blue colour—the lotion and ointments I used were not calculated to make it blister, but it did blister, and then the skin came off, and the blueness was gone.

The lotion was a mixture of lime water and linseed oil.

Smithies stated that when he had started an early morning fire for cooking purposes with shavings, it had got out of control. His household goods and the stock of his tobacconist's shop were reported to be insured for £700. He was found guilty of murder and sentenced to death (*OB*, July 1832: pp. 593–610).

An incendiary device employing gunpowder having been found, the evidence for gunpowder residue in or on Smithies' skin was an important part of the case. The surgeon's experience, unlike that of the apothecary, with this kind of "tattooing" from a powder explosion was admittedly limited, and the defense made the most of the situation. Yet it also seems quite possible that particles of residue were driven only lightly into the outer layers of the skin and were lost when these layers were sloughed during healing. When Smithies was hurt, the powder would have exploded in the open space of the vault, not while confined as in a gun barrel or as in a shot hole in a mine. The force of the blast would thus have been relatively low, and the penetrating power of particles of gunpowder would not have been great.

Spontaneous human combustion and the "preternatural combustibility" of the human body were accepted as rare but perfectly possible phenomena by some forensic and other medical experts, even in the eighteenth and nineteenth centuries (Adelson, 1952; 1974: pp. 613–15). According to the first of these strange and unfounded superstitions, on rare occasions a human body could spontaneously burst into flames and rapidly be consumed, leaving a few ashes and an evil smell. Nearby objects were almost untouched. "Preternatural combustibility" referred to a condition in which, it was alleged, a human being, set on fire by even the smallest flame, would be rapidly and completely incinerated. In neither case was any fuel required.

Ryan wrote in 1831 in his *Manual of Medical Jurisprudence:*

> It is now admitted on the continent of Europe, though disbelieved in these countries [the British Isles], that spontaneous combustion is possible, though its cause is as yet inexplicable. It is said to occur most commonly to aged females, who have long indulged in the abuse of alcoholic potations. Generally speaking, some manner of ignition, as a lighted candle, a pipe, &c has been found near the remains of the body; but cases are attested in which no igneous substances were discovered. (p. 218)

Ogston, almost fifty years later, gave it as his opinion that spontaneous human combustion "may now be safely set aside as inadmissible," while human preternatural combustibility "is also believed by our best writers on medical jurisprudence to carry with it its own condemnation . . . . The question . . . is one which I think should still be considered *sub judice*" (1878: pp. 463–64).

FIREARM WOUNDS

Conventional gunshot wounds seem to have presented no great challenge to the careful forensic medical observer. For example, an intruder was fatally wounded in the head when a revolver was fired in the dark to frighten him. The bullet was recognized to have "marks upon it that could not have been made in penetrating the skull . . . . the shape of the bullet is exceedingly distorted and altered—if fired point blank, it would have gone through his skull, if some substance had not intercepted it—my notion is, that it struck against some hard substance, and reflected [ricocheted] on the body of the man." A police officer found a fresh chip from a brick in a wall in the presumed line of fire (*OB,* July 1865: pp. 228–32).

The significance of the spreading pattern of shot discharged from a gun was recognized. A woman was killed with a pistol loaded with fine lead shot. The autopsy surgeon noted that "the Pistol must be held quite close to the Body, to make such a Wound as this; for which I have two Reasons; the first is, if the Pistol had been at some Distance from the Body, the Shot would have separated, whereas, they all went in at one Orifice: My other Reason is, because the Lips of the Wound were actually burnt with the Powder" (*OB,* Dec. 1739: pp. 4–5).

STARVATION

The notorious murder trial of the Stauntons in 1877 disclosed a homicide allegedly by starvation. The facts, briefly told, were that Harriet Richardson, a thirty-six-year-old woman "of weakened intellect," had married Louis Staunton against her mother's wishes. The daughter had an estate of over £3,000. Her twenty-three-year-old husband was penniless. Following the wedding the mother was unable to communicate with Harriet or locate her. When, by chance, word of her death two years later reached a relative, he managed to locate the doctor who had signed the death certificate. Foul play was suspected, the coroner was notified, and the body was exhumed. During the inquest it developed that the mentally deficient Harriet had for some months been held a virtual prisoner by her husband, his brother, the brother's wife, and the latter's sister. All four were indicted for murder.

At the trial the principal medical issue was whether Harriet had died of disease or of starvation and neglect during her imprisonment.

Dr. Longrigg, the physician who signed the death certificate, had specified cerebral disease as the primary, and apoplexy as the secondary, cause of death. He admitted that he had seen Harriet only once, and then only for a few minutes when she was dying, and that he had made his diagnosis largely on the basis of information supplied by the prisoners. The autopsy surgeons reported that the body was emaciated, filthy, and verminous. The uterus was enlarged; the other internal organs were essentially normal except for some congestion. (Not long before her death, Harriet had given birth to a son, who soon succumbed.) Poisoning was suspected, but analysis of various viscera and also of the stomach contents disclosed no toxic substance.

The six medical witnesses for the prosecution agreed in general, although not in all particulars, that Harriet Staunton had died because of starvation and not, as had been suggested by counsel for the accused, from diabetes, Addison's disease, or tuberculous meningitis. Two medical witnesses for the defense asserted that death was due to the latter and that the emaciation could have been secondary to that disease. Their opinion was supported by a pathologist who had seen the records although not the body.

The judge's summing-up for the jury reveals his bias:

> His lordship then dealt with the medical evidence, observing—The organs of the deceased appeared to be in a healthy condition, except for the emaciation. You have heard a medical witness cross examined. *But why make these examinations in pursuit of something you have no reason to believe existed?* [Italics added.] A sufficient cause for death presented itself on examination, and the tubercular deposits were not considered of importance.
>
> There was nothing, his lordship said, in his judgment to show that death arose from this tubercular meningitis, or any other such disease. (Atlay, 1911: p. 279)

All four defendants were found guilty. On 26 September they heard the judge sentence them to die on 16 October.

The *Lancet* for 6 October carried a lengthy article by Dr. Greenfield, the defense witness. He discussed the medical evidence in detail, concluding in part:

> So far, then, there seems to be in the medical statements as to facts no particle of evidence that the emaciation was due to want of food, and still less to wilful starvation. On the other hand, there is evidence that the immediate cause of death was an acute disease, nor is there anything to show that it was induced or increased by starvation or neglect . . . .
>
> It is only right to add that . . . . the tubercular nature of the nodules seems now to be pretty certainly established. (Greenfield, 1877)

An editorial in the same issue of the journal entirely supported the views of Greenfield and strongly attacked the interpretation of testimony by Mr. Justice Hawkins, the judge, in his summing-up. Said the *Lancet*:

> Our contention is simply and expressly that the conviction is bad in fact and therefore, we presume, bad in law. The judge left the case to the jury on the allegation of murder by starvation. We have no hesitation in affirming that the fundamental proposition of this court, namely, that the deceased died of starvation, is not only unproved, but entirely unsupported by the evidence . . . . it must obviously be impossible to prove *murder* by starvation without first showing *death* by starvation . . . . it is clear there was disease, and the life of Harriet Staunton was not therefore sacrificed by want of food alone . . . . What we desire to place on record is a strong belief that the indications offered by a dead body imperfectly examined have been misinterpreted, and an inference drawn which the facts do not warrant, but which, on the contrary, they controvert. (*Lancet,* 1877)

Seven hundred medical men, among them Sir William Jenner, physician to the queen, set their names to a memorial proposed by the editors of the *Lancet*. The document asserted, in effect, that Mrs. Staunton had died of cerebral disease and that this had caused her emaciation. The press joined in with a vigorous attack on the verdict, as did the novelist Charles Reade. The Home Secretary reopened the case, and the death penalty was remitted on 14 October. After another two weeks Alice Rhodes, one of the four defendants, was pardoned, and the sentences of the other three were commuted to penal servitude for life (*OB,* Sept. 1877: pp. 327–47, 365–66, 386–93; Atlay, 1911: pp. 1–29, 279–87, 291, 317–25).

Woodman and Tidy's *Forensic Medicine and Toxicology,* published the year of the Staunton trial, devotes a number of pages to starvation, malnourishment, the requirements for a proper diet, and related matters, but does not discuss emaciation caused by disease. Taylor's *Medical Jurisprudence* (1856), however, after describing post-mortem appearances in starvation, warns that they "should be accompanied by an otherwise healthy state of the body; since, as it is well known, they may be produced by many organic diseases, and death may be thus due to disease, and not to the mere privation of food" (p. 622).

PUBLIC NUISANCE

Early in the nineteenth century London and other English cities still had no central administrative mechanism for the protection of the public health (Rosen, 1958: p. 160). Recognizing the problem, Farr's *Elements of Medical Jurisprudence* listed numerous steps that should be taken to preserve the health of the community, including the protection of air, water, and food from contamination, proper shelter for foundlings and the insane, the regulation of apothecaries and midwives, the prevention of contagious disease, and so on (pp. 72–80). John Gordon Smith divided forensic medicine into four areas; one of them encompassed "whatever regards the preservation of the public health; as the proper regulations in times of public sickness, the administration of public institutions for the cure of diseases, public nuisances, and many subjects of the last [sic] importance, forming that conspicuous department, termed *Medical Police*" (1821: p. 13). Some fifty-four pages of Traill's *Outlines of a Course of Lectures on Medical Jurisprudence* were devoted to "Medical Police" (1841: pp. 180–234). One concern was the purity of the atmosphere, although only in terms of nitrogen, oxygen, carbonic acid, and "aqueous vapour" (p. 213). Alfred Swaine Taylor went much farther, discussing at some length the dangers of industrial air pollutants including carbonic acid, charcoal vapor, and various gaseous sulfur compounds (1856: pp. 595–613).

The aspirations of these and other writers in the field of legal medicine for the promotion of community well-being are commendable, but prosecution of offenders against public health and safety was not frequent as far as the Old Bailey was concerned. The public health activities of forensic medical experts were pretty much limited to testimony in a modest number of trials of persons charged with mistreatment of mental patients, with child abuse, or, in the 1860s and 1870s, with creation of certain public nuisances and hazards. Active in the attack on the latter was Dr. Henry Letheby, medical officer of health, food analyst, and chief examiner of illuminating gas for the City of London.

Letheby gave testimony in a startling public health and safety case in 1855. A clergyman, master of Merchant Taylors' School near Thames Street and the river, complained bitterly of offensive odors reaching his home and the adjoining school from a nearby warehouse. The smell was worst when the warehousemen were "mixing of some spirit or other—I have seen the mixing going on in the street—they transfer the spirit from one vessel to another called the tarboy [carboy]. . . I perceived on my premises there was a very noxious smell of this naphtha . . . . I and my wife and family sleep on my premises, and a good many boarders—I now have sixteen." The neighbors supported the clergyman's complaint, identifying the odor as that of "naphtha." One of them added that "there was great danger—one night I went into my yard with a candle at 12 o'clock, and it [the atmosphere] caught light—there was a blue light around it."

Then the medical men testified:

> DR. ALFRED SWAINE TAYLOR. I am a doctor of medicine, and fellow of the Royal Society, and have very extensive practice as a chemist. On the 19th October I went to examine the defendant's premises—I perceived . . . a smell which I immediately recognised as wood naphtha [wood alcohol and acetone]—it was strong . . . . I found wood naphtha stored there with other things—the defendants said the wood naphtha amounted to about 5,000 gallons—it was in tins . . . . there was spirits of wine [alcohol] . . . . there were two large vats for mixing this naphtha with spirits of wine . . . . nausea, headache, and giddiness are such symptoms as naphtha, mixed with air, would produce—it is decidedly narcotic . . . . is very inflammable . . . . in hot weather it would be very dangerous to bring any light in connection with it . . . . if any fire were to take place in the neighbourhood, it would be a most dreadful explosion, I think more dangerous than gunpowder . . . . 5,000 gallons would have the effect of burning down a large part of London.
>
> DR. HENRY LETHEBY. I examined the defendant's premises on the 24th Nov.—there were about 800 gallons of naphtha there . . . . it is very volatile, indeed, it is very inflammable—if there were any fire in the neighbourhood . . . . I found no lights were used on the premises. (*OB,* Nov. 1855: pp. 237–44)

Such appalling hazards could exist because, it seems, there were no laws regarding the storage and handling of dangerous chemicals. Gunpowder, incidentally, was also kept in quantity in the metropolis, as became evident when there was a fatal explosion in a fireworks factory (Forbes, 1977b).

Another threat to the public health was the uncontrolled sale of spoiled, diseased, and filthy meat. Slaughterhouses were not effectively regulated. Meat was not marked to show its quality; street vendors were not licensed. Spoiled meat, disdained by well-to-do persons, was readily sold at lower prices to the poor who, able to afford little protein at any cost, could scarcely be particular (F. B. Smith, 1979: pp. 203–07). In 1860 a campaign to control the slaughter of unhealthy animals in the City of London was undertaken. The *Lancet* reported that an inspection of abattoirs in the City resulted in the seizure of 1,192 pounds of meat considered unfit for human consumption; all of it was destroyed (Unwholesome, 1860). The response of some butchers was to have meat shipped in by train from slaughterhouses outside London (F. B. Smith: p. 204).

The *Lancet* continued its campaign and in February 1861 was able to commend the Sewers Committee of the Corporation of London for the first successful prosecution in many years of a butcher for selling rotten meat, in this case mutton.[1] Dr. Letheby testified in court "that if such meat got into the animal body in a partially cooked state it produced either low fever or violent vomiting and purging" (More food, 1861).

In April of the same year another butcher was prosecuted for unlawfully exposing for sale five hundred pounds of beef unfit for human consumption. It had been shipped into London from a slaughterhouse thirty-four miles away. After the inspectors and others had given their evidence, Letheby testified that in his judgment the meat "was not fit for human food—it was from a very diseased animal . . . . the animal had an epidemic inflammatory affection of the lung." The defense alleged that the cow in question was healthy but had broken a rib while on a train. The prisoner was found guilty and was sentenced to two weeks in confinement (*OB,* April 1861: pp. 519–29).

Another offender was tried on a similar charge the next month. After testimony by two inspectors of meat at Newgate market, both employed by the Commissioners of Sewers of the Corporation of London, Letheby again came to the stand. He stated that these beef carcasses also showed the signs of lung disease.

It turned out that the meat had been shipped into London in a hamper by train. It also was established that the defendant had been a witness for the defense in the diseased meat case a month earlier, a fact confirmed by the official shorthand writer to the court:

> I took a note of the evidence he gave—I have those notes here, also the printed report of the evidence—that printed report is a correct transcript of my notes in a narrative form—I have examined it and it is correct.
>
> (*The evidence given by the defendant on the trial of Spencer was here read from the Sessions Paper.*)[2]

The accused meat dealer was found guilty and sentenced to two months in prison (*OB,* May 1861: pp. 39–45). There was a similar trial later in the same month (*OB,* May 1861: pp. 55–59).

The campaign continued. In November 1862 the *Lancet* quoted at

1. That the enforcement of laws regulating the sale of meat was in the hands of this committee was an indication of the fragmented administration of public health measures.

2. Thus the *Sessions Papers* still constituted the official court record.

length from a recent report by Letheby, in particular giving disgusting details about the manufacture of sausages at Cow-cross, just outside of London and therefore beyond the City's control. City butchers complained of discriminatory practices:

> In like manner, at Whitechapel it is a common practice with some of the butchers, who are outside the City boundaries, to traffic in diseased meat; and the City butchers and salesmen complain that they have not the same chance for the disposal of inferior meat which their neighbours have, and the rigorous supervision of the City is unjust to them. Only last week the carcasses of several bullocks, about a dozen or so, that had died on ship board, were sold in Whitechapel. Meat of this description is disposed of to the poor at night, when it passes for wholesome meat, and it realizes from a penny to five farthings a pound. (Diseased, 1862, *Lancet*)

Letheby carried on with support from the *Lancet* for several years and there were additional trials of unscrupulous meat dealers at the Old Bailey.

MALINGERING

Malingering was a rare but not unknown offense in the courtroom. Its detection required an expert witness. For example, Thomas Cinnamon was put on trial in 1719 for theft:

> The Prisoner was brought to the Bar appearing in a very weak and helpless Condition, as if not able to walk, or help himself, and with a Rug hanging over his Shoulder, under pretence of being in a Salivation, and Tongue so swelled he could not speak[3] and being arraigned supported himself upon the Bar, and for a considerable Time would not by any means plead to his Indictment tho threatened with the Press,[4] till the Court ordering a Surgeon to be called, who examining his Mouth &c. found it was more obstinacy than inability, which when he had deposed in Court, the Prisoner was presently cured of his dumbness and pleading to his Indictment took his Tryal.

Cinnamon was found guilty and was sentenced to death (*OB,* Jan. 1719: pp. 1–2).

3. At this time various mercury compounds were taken internally in the treatment of venereal disease. When the bodily concentration of the metal rose high enough, the patient salivated profusely. Chronic mercury poisoning could also cause inflammation and swelling of the mucosa of the mouth.

4. The torture of pressing, or *peine forte et dure,* could still be legally applied at this time to try to force an accused person to plead or place himself on trial.

A French prisoner, François Mercier, was indicted for murder: *"When the Prisoner was set to the bar and arraigned, he stood mute; therefore the Court directed the sheriff to return a jury to enquire whether he stood mute through obstinacy, or by the visitation of God."* The jury was so sworn. Then four witnesses testified that they had not only heard the prisoner speak but that the night before the trial he had carried on a conversation in English. But just before he entered the courtroom, they said, he could only mumble:

> At this point one of the jurymen made a request. "My Lord, the Jury would be glad to have the opinion of some medical gentleman whether the prisoner may not have taken some medicine that might have produced the effect to take away his speech." Mr. Thomas Ogle, a surgeon present in court, was asked to examine the prisoner. Ogle could not decide whether the accused was able to speak.
>
> *The Jury, after consulting together for a short time, found that he stood mute fraudulently, and obstinately, and not by the providence of God.*
>
> *Upon which Mr. Justice Aston . . . immediately passed sentence upon him, That he should be executed on Monday, December 8, and his body be afterwards dissected and anatomized.—Which sentence was accordingly executed upon him.* (*OB*, Dec. 1777: pp. 18–19; Gentleman's, 1777)

According to the *New Newgate Calendar,* Mercier had earlier confessed to robbing and murdering his employer (Knapp and Baldwin, 1820?: 3, 396–98).

MALPRACTICE AND QUACKERY

London of course had its share of quacks, who treated their patients without adequate medical education and depended on experience, quick wits, and effrontery. Misdeeds brought several of these individuals to the Old Bailey, particularly in the first half of the nineteenth century. When a patient of Edwin Martin Van Butchell[5] died, it was revealed at the inquest that he had treated a rectal stricture in a male patient by probing the canal with a long ivory rod. The patient's subsequent history and autopsy revealed all the signs of a rectal per-

5. The quack's father, also an empiric, had studied anatomy with John Hunter. He practiced dentistry with success, then acquired a reputation for making trusses and treating anal fistulas. Flocks of patients responded to his florid advertisements. Van Butchell traveled about the London streets on a pony painted purple, brandishing a bleached human femur. Following the death of his first wife, he kept her embalmed body for years in a glass case in his parlor. It was only after the empiric remarried that the departure of the first Mrs. Van Butchell was completed.

foration. At the trial a medical witness asserted on the stand that to probe the rectum "no properly educated surgeon would use a straight unyielding instrument" like the empiric's ivory rod. But he and his patient were alone when the examination was made, and it could not be proved that Van Butchell had produced the fatal injury.

Mr. Baron Hullock, the judge, learning that the prosecution had no stronger evidence, gave it as his opinion that no case had been made out. He then rendered an important judgment regarding medical malpractice:

> if such an indictment could be supported, in the total absence of all evidence of want of skill or neglect, because an operation failed, the consequences would be most serious, whether the operation was performed by a regular or an irregular surgeon; and surely it would be most unjust to prosecute a man who might be a skilful and clever practitioner, upon the unsuccessful result of a dangerous operation, because he was not licensed, and not fortunate enough to possess the sanction and authority of a certain body in this town.

This last was a reference to the Royal College of Surgeons, of which Van Butchell was not a licentiate. The justice continued, asserting that if "such a doctrine could be maintained, very many persons in remote parts would be unable to procure any assistance; for who would exercise their best skill, of whatever quality it might be, if in the case of failure they were to be subjected to an indictment for murder or manslaughter?" Justice Hullock declared, in the words of the *London Medical Gazette,* "that it made no difference whether the practitioner was regular or irregular; and he added that there was no instance on record in which either had been tried for manslaughter in consequence of real or alleged bad practice" (Trial, 1829). The jury was directed to find a verdict of not guilty, and decided accordingly.

Thus Van Butchell seems to have been the first regular or irregular practitioner to be tried in England for manslaughter resulting from malpractice. The *London Medical Gazette,* while it could not approve of his dangerous incompetence, was relieved at the verdict: "no one practicing surgery according to the best of his skill, is committing an "unlawful act," and therefore he cannot be guilty of manslaughter . . . . People do not make very nice distinctions between regular and irregular practitioners; and if the accused in this instance had been convicted, we should soon have had abundance of such prosecutions."[6]

John St. John Long, another quack, treated a variety of diseases by

6. *OB,* June 1829: pp. 598–600; Trial, 1829; Forbes, 1976b.

applying an unidentified escharotic or caustic ointment to the skin. The resulting sore was then anointed with a lotion and bandaged with a cabbage leaf. In addition the patient was instructed to inhale a particular but unidentified vapor. One of Long's patients, Catherine Cashin, was said by him to be suffering from pulmonary tuberculosis. The lesion he produced on her back, although praised by the quack as beneficial, spread and became progressively more inflamed and painful. Sir Benjamin Brodie, the prominent London surgeon who was eventually called in by the patient's family, testified at Long's trial for manslaughter to observing a reddened area "as large as the whole of a common plate." In the center was a necrotic "spot as big as the palm of my hand." Miss Cashin, very ill by the time Brodie saw her, died the next morning.

Apparently a partial autopsy was done. Except for the large lesion, which was found to involve the spinal meninges, no appearance of disease was noted. The prisoner denied any responsibility for the death.

There appeared for the defense an extraordinary procession of thirty character witnesses, including three members of the nobility, a colonel, a lieutenant general, and the Surgeon General of Jamaica. All had been Long's patients or were relatives of patients, and all testified to his "skill, attention, and humanity." The jury, not impressed, found him guilty (*OB,* Oct. 1830: pp. 856–62).

Three months later Long was back at the Old Bailey, this time for the death by manslaughter of Colin Compbell Loyd, wife of a captain in the Royal Navy. Because of a cold, she had at Long's direction applied "a small blister" to her throat. Three days later, the quack himself treated her. Soon the lesion was badly inflamed, suppurating, painful, and widespread. Long saw her again and ordered the dressings replaced with cabbage leaves. The patient's condition worsened. Brodie and another surgeon visited her, but she died of a generalized infection a month and a day after her first visit to the quack. An autopsy revealed that, except for the lesion and a slight narrowing of the esophagus, "the whole body, both internal and external, was in a very healthy state."

The prisoner conducted much of his own defense, seeking to shift the blame, claiming that his directions for the patient had not been followed, and alleging persecution. His closing appeal displayed the eloquence that had won him many a patient:

> I leave my case in the hands of a British Judge and Jury; how many medical men might be brought here if answerable in this way? Who

> would attend you, gentlemen, if ill tomorrow? I am told I stand here on the same footing as a member of the College of Physicians—I have as much liberty to practice as they have, provided I have done no harm; this is nothing but a persecution against me, because I have discovered a remedy for the care of consumptions—the prevention of small pox—the removal of the gout—and of insanity.

Again Long was followed to the stand by a procession of character witnesses. The twenty-six individuals included merchants, a solicitor, and a Member of Parliament. This time the quack was found not guilty (*OB,* Jan. 1831: pp. 283–91).[7]

PHYSICAL EVIDENCE

Careful examination of the scene of a crime and of the clothing and other possessions of the victim, as well as of the body of the deceased, sometimes yielded useful information. A member of the Bow Street patrol noticed blood on the glove of a murder suspect. It was then observed that a square piece of cloth had been torn from the bottom of the suspect's trouser leg. Later a blood stained cloth fragment was found at the death scene; the fragment fitted exactly the defect in the trousers (*OB,* Jan. 1833: pp. 118–26).

In another homicide case the print of a boot was noticed in a pool of blood; "from the direction of the footprint the foot would be coming from the room." The board bearing the print was removed as evidence. Then a bloody boot was found hidden in a dustbin. The boot, including the pattern of its nails, exactly fitted the print on the board. A package of valuables stolen at the time of the murder was also recovered. The bundle was tied with a cloth tape. The latter matched a piece of tape found in the suspect's room. Each piece had thirty-three strands, and drapers on the coroner's jury agreed that the two pieces were identical (*OB,* Oct. 1860: pp. 769–805).

The science of blood chemistry developed very slowly. For a long time it was not possible, for example, to determine whether a blood

7. A few months later he triumphed in yet another legal encounter. The *Gentleman's Magazine* noted: "An action was tried June 14 in the Common Pleas, brought by St. John Long, the *medical* gentleman whose name has of late been tolerably familiar to the public ear, against a pamphleteer of the name of Chubb, residing in Holywell-street, Strand, for a libel, purporting to be a life of the nostrum-monger, in which he was rather roughly handled. The Jury, after remaining out several hours, returned a verdict for the plaintiff—damages 100 *l.*! (*Gentleman's,* 1831b: pp. 101, 553–54).

sample was of human or animal origin. At the trial of Frederick and Maria Manning in 1849 for the murder of Patrick O'Connor, a chemist described the tests he had performed to determine whether spots on a garment actually were those of blood:

> I cut out the stained portion of the dress and cut it into several slips, which I suspended one after another in a small quantity of distilled water; they imparted their colour to the water—it was a smoky red colour, from which I afterwards obtained a precipitate indicating albumen, one of the constituents of blood . . . . there is no direct chemical process which will identify blood stains . . . . I did not examine it by the microscope. (*OB,* Oct. 1849: pp. 654–79)

The chemist's tests obviously were far from definitive.

Microscopic examination of a spot on a pencil case in 1860 led an expert witness to state that

> in my judgment that spot was blood—a microscope is an infallible test as far as regards the proof of blood . . . .
>
> MR. SERJEANT PARRY. *Q.* Unfortunately at present there is no test by which you can detect human blood from other blood, is there? *A.* No. (*OB,* Oct. 1860: pp. 769–805)

On an evening in July 1864 a passenger on a train leaving London was startled to discover blood in a first-class compartment. The guard was called, the compartment was locked, and the carriage was removed from the train and held for investigation. Also on that evening a body was found beside the train's right of way.

As a result of much police work, Franz Muller was arrested on the ship *Victoria* when it arrived in New York on 24 August, and was brought back to London. He was charged with the murder of the dead traveler, Thomas Briggs, and was tried at the Old Bailey. Medical witnesses who had performed a post-mortem examination of the victim described multiple head wounds and fractures, evidently produced in part by blows from a blunt instrument and in part by the fall from the train to the ground. Dr. Henry Letheby's testimony regarding the blood stains in the railway carriage revealed some advances in forensic medical science:

> I observed blood on two of the cushions . . . . it had all the characteristics of human blood—I have measured the globules of the blood, and believe it to be human blood . . . . There was blood on the glass immediately over the cushion—it was blood having all the characteristics of human blood—it was blood that had been living when it came on the glass, from the coagulum in it, and it contained also particles of brain matter . . . . if a person had been sitting on that part

> of the carriage, and had been struck on the left side of his head as he was leaning his head against the glass, that effect might have been produced.

Letheby's "globules" were red blood corpuscles (*OB,* Oct. 1864: pp. 461–504).

The 1877 edition of Woodman and Tidy's textbook gave the diameters of the dried corpuscles of a large number of vertebrates from fish to man as a basis for determining the source of such cells, but for technical reasons the accurate identification of human red corpuscles by this method seems unlikely. The guaiac test for identification of blood as such, also described by Woodman and Tidy, is much more reliable. Their chapter on blood stains is concluded with three questions that may be put to the expert medical witness:

> 1) Was the blood human?
> 2) From what part of the body was it derived? and,
> 3) What is the probable age of the stain?
>
> To these questions, as a rule, you had better confess your inability to reply. Never venture rash answers. The replies can, save in a few exceptional cases, be little else than guesses; and it is dangerous in the extreme to guess in the witness box. (pp. 520–28)

Benjamin Hooker, a surgeon, in 1760 made a thorough examination of the body of a woman found dead in a pond with a ligature drawn tight round her neck. Her head and face were bruised and lacerated and there was hemorrhage under the scalp, but the skull was not fractured. Had she died of the blow to the head, or drowning, or strangulation? Hooker shrewdly concluded that "she could not die by drowning, for her mouth was full of blood [from the head injuries]; upon removing her garters, there were no black marks, as under the ferretting[8] about her neck which confirm'd me in it that she was strangled" (*OB,* Sept. 1760: pp. 288–96).

We can reconstruct Hooker's reasoning. Blood would not have filled the mouth after death, as bleeding virtually stops after the heart has ceased to contract. If death had been due to drowning in the pond, the airway would have been blocked with water, not blood. Loose constriction of the legs by the garters produced no visible skin changes, but the pressure of the violently applied ferretting broke small subcutaneous blood vessels, and hemorrhage from the latter left black marks, that is, ecchymoses or bruises. Since bleeding occurs only during life, the ferretting was applied before death. Had the head

8. A kind of strong tape made of cotton or silk.

injuries been inflicted after strangling—an unlikely event—hemorrhage into the mouth would not have occurred. So the victim was struck on the head, then strangled, then thrown dead into the pond.

A man was punched and then struck twice on the head with a long stick, the handle of a bricklayer's server.[9] The victim died of his injuries. When a police officer

> found the stick it was in the state it is now in, with a few drops of blood on it, and the server had some hair on it; it appears to me to be human hair—it adhered to it quite close, as if it had been a blow . . . .
>
> *Q*. Have you had the stick ever since? *A*. No, it has been locked up in the superintendent's room—we have not washed it . . . . human hair is sometimes used with mortar, I believe, for a shift[10]—the server is used to scoop mortar; it had been in mortar . . . . the hair was on the edge of it; I did not compare the hair with anything.

In other words, was the human hair on the server from the mortar or from the head of the victim? The question was not resolved (*OB*, May 1831: pp. 527–31). Taylor some years later pointed out that hairs found on a murder weapon could be of either human or animal origin but gave no clue as to how the distinction could be made (1856: p. 213).

A physician and surgeon in 1860 conducted an autopsy of an old woman who had died of severe head injuries. They also examined a bloody

> boot with a powerful magnifying glass—I found one hair between the welt and the sole in this broken side, the best part of of it was packed within the boot; I found another hair on the surface, and a third here—I am of opinion that they were human hairs . . . . part of them were cut up to put under the microscope.
>
> COURT. *Q*. Do you say that they are certainly human hairs? *A*. Certainly—I ascertained that by means of the microscope—my experience enables me to say that they are human hairs—I could tell what colour they were—they were much the same colour as Mrs. Emsley's [the victim's] hair . . . . I compared the hairs with what I actually took from her head. (*OB*, Oct. 1860: pp. 769–805)

Note that the witness was sure that the hair was human but not that it was identical with hair from the victim's head. By 1877, however, Woodman and Tidy were able to describe many microscopic details of human and animal hair (pp. 497–501).

9. A small spade used by plasterers and others.

10. That is, as a substitute for the animal hair that was sometimes mixed with mortar.

IDENTIFICATION OF THE ACCUSED

With the exception of the *Old Bailey Sessions Papers,* official records of London criminal court trials were limited, consisting mostly of lists of names, dates, offenses, verdicts, and sentences. Also lacking was detailed verbal identification of prisoners.[11] The Bertillon system, fingerprinting, personal photographs, and organized detailed central records all were to come later. In the courtroom, the judge was dependent on his own recollection or that of a court officer or policeman as to whether a prisoner at the bar had previously been convicted (Rumbelow, 1971: p. 178):[12]

> JOSEPH DALTON (*City-policeman,* No. 366). I produce a certificate of Carney's former conviction (*read, Convicted 6th of January, 1845, of larceny and confined six months.*) I was present at the trial—the prisoner is the person. (*OB,* Nov. 1845: p. 63)
>
> JONATHAN WHICHER. I produce a certificate—(*Read: "Central Criminal Court, Jan. 1850, James Hughes, convicted of housebreaking, and transported for ten Years."*)
>
> JOSEPH METTAM. I was present at the trial—Hopkins is the man—I was the prosecutor in the case. (*OB,* April 1856: p. 794)

Note the latter prisoner's change of name.

Incidental use of a photograph for identification of a suspect was mentioned in the *Sessions Papers* in 1866 and again in 1868 (*OB,* Sept. 1866: pp. 414–32; Aug. 1868: pp. 314–22). Systematic identification of criminals by their photographs apparently was first suggested in England in 1894 by a committee appointed by the Secretary of State for the Home Department (Glaister, 1928b: pp. 422–23).

Physical evidence and details of personal appearance were important in the solution of three sensational London homicides.

11. English law enforcement officers were seriously hampered by the lack of a system for regularly preparing the descriptions of wanted criminals and for circulating this information to the appropriate authorities. In an effort to overcome these difficulties, the magistrate Sir John Fielding in 1772 had publicized his General Preventative Plan. It provided for the submission of written descriptions of wanted persons to a central file in Fielding's office in Bow Street and for the publication of the descriptions in newspapers (Styles, 1983: pp. 136–41). But the *Sessions Papers* do not indicate that the courts grappled with the problem of prisoner identification through written descriptions.

12. The blind magistrate, Sir John Fielding, was alleged to have known three thousand offenders by their voices.

THE COOK MURDER

Problems in the identification of the bodies of two rather similar elderly women, one of them a murder victim, arose during a police investigation. The inquiry resulted in January 1832 in the trial of Elizabeth Ross, alias Cook, aged thirty-eight, and her husband, Edward Cook, for the death of their lodger, Caroline Walsh, aged eighty-four years. This was a case of "burking," homicide to procure a body for sale to the anatomists. The murder followed by about a month the execution of Bishop and Williams for the burking death of the "Italian boy" (chapter 3).[13] The Cook case added new fuel to public outrage stirred by the earlier crimes and helped to bring about the reforms embodied in the Warburton Anatomy Act, passed by Parliament later in 1832.

The Cooks' trial began with the testimony of their son, aged twelve. He told how on the afternoon of Friday, 19 August 1831, one Caroline Walsh, a poor street vendor, came to lodge with the Cooks in their single room. That evening she drank some coffee they offered and promptly fell asleep on the bed. Then, asserted the son, as he and his father looked on, Mrs. Cook smothered the old woman by pressing her hands on the victim's mouth and chest. Later on Mrs. Cook carried the body to the basement, put it in a sack, and hid it under the stairs, where her son discovered it the next morning. That night, Saturday, she put the sack and its contents on her shoulder and bore them away, confiding to her son on Sunday morning that she had delivered them to the London Hospital. Undoubtedly she had then sold the corpse, probably to the beadle of the dissecting rooms.

Ann Buton, the granddaughter of Caroline Walsh, the victim, followed the Cooks' son to the witness stand. The murdered woman, said Mrs. Buton, was of Irish birth, tall and vigorous for her years, and earned her living as a street pedlar, selling tapes, laces, thread, and the like. Ann Buton and her sister had seen their grandmother on the afternoon of 19 August, the day of her death, and were able to describe her clothing in detail.

The beadle of the Parish of Allhallows Staining, not far from where the Cooks lived, told how late on Saturday, the night after the

13. The first known instance of smothering a victim to procure a body for sale occurred in 1752, when two Edinburgh nursemaids killed a boy aged eight or nine by this method and sold the corpse to medical students (Guttmacher, 1935: p. 392).

murder, he had found *another* tall elderly Irish woman sitting on a doorstep. She was Catherine Walchman, or Welch, also an itinerant street vendor, and she was sick, in pain, and unable to walk. He carried her to the watchhouse. There she was seen by a surgeon, who discovered an old fracture of the hip. Exhausted, filthy, and homeless, she was moved to the Hoxton poorhouse. The woman stayed there four or five days, then was taken to the London Hospital, where she died on 3 September. Her clothes, ragged and verminous, were burned. The nurse who prepared the body for burial noticed several significant anatomical details about which she later testified.

On Saturday morning, 20 August, Mrs. Buton returned and found Mrs. Cook alone in her room. Caroline Walsh, said the landlady, had just gone out. The Buton woman became suspicious and suggested that she and Mrs. Cook go out for a "drop of gin." Liquor loosened the murderer's tongue a bit, but not enough. Ann Buton searched for several weeks for her grandmother, visiting hospitals, jails, and poorhouses. As a result of her inquiries at the London Hospital, the grave of Catherine Welch was opened. This was sometime in September or early October. The beadle of the dissecting rooms at the London Hospital was later to testify that he had been present at both the burial and the exhumation of the old woman; his presence implies that the body had been dissected. In any case, Ann Buton, also an observer when the grave was opened, was positive from the appearance of the teeth, feet, skin, and hair that the corpse was *not* that of her grandmother, Caroline Walsh. A nurse identified the body as that of Caroline Welch.

All three of the Cooks were arrested. Two police constables transported the family in a coach to Newgate Prison on 22 December. One of the officers described their conversation en route. Edward Cook

> said I [Constable James Lea] had had a great deal of trouble in this business—I said Yes: the woman said, "With all your trouble you have not found the old woman's body". . . . she said, "That was the old woman that was taken to Bethnal-green workhouse."
>
> *Q*. You mean Mrs. Walsh? *A*. Yes, she alluded to her; the man [Edward Cook] corrected her, and said it was Hoxton workhouse—she said, "That was the woman that died in the London-hospital."

Clearly the Cook woman had heard how Catherine Welch had been picked up in the street in a neighboring parish, twenty-four hours after the disappearance of Caroline Walsh, and also how the Welch woman had been taken to the workhouse, had died in London

Hospital, and had been buried there. What Mrs. Cook did not know about was the exhumation of the body of Catherine Welch.

After the unexplained delay in beginning an investigation into the disappearance of Caroline Walsh, the police had been hard at work, and a formidable body of evidence had been gathered by the time the trial of the Cooks began. Several surgeons and nurses who had attended Catherine Welch in the London Hospital testified as to her condition and physical appearance while there. A pawnbroker and various old clothes dealers told of acquiring a woman's garments and a supply of threads, laces, and tapes from Mrs. Cook. Ann Buton was able positively to identify the clothes as those worn by her grandmother. Significant evidence elicited in court may be compared:

Caroline Walsh	*Catherine Welch*
Grandmother of Ann Buton.	Family unknown.
Came from Kilkenny, Ireland.	Came from Waterford, Ireland.
Eighty-four years old.	Sixty-one years old.
Sold tapes, laces, thread from basket in street.	Sold matches from basket in street.
Tall, hearty, upright, clean.	Tall, feeble, stooped, filthy.
Light skin.	Very dark skin.
No fractures.	Broken hip.
Front teeth "good" in both jaws.	Front teeth all missing.
Toes all straight, no deformities.	Two toes overlapped, bunions, corns.
Wore black stuff [worsted] gown, black willow bonnet, gray knitted stockings, men's shoes, light blue shawl with distinctive stain. Most of these were identified as having been sold by Mrs. Cook.	Wore blue gown, black silk bonnet; stockings were not knitted.

On 6 January Edward Cook was found not guilty. His wife was convicted of murder (*OB,* Jan. 1832: pp. 146–54). She was hanged three days later (Domestic, 1831: pp. 461, 643).

Unfortunately, neither the *Sessions Papers* nor the *Gentleman's Magazine* answered two important questions: What happened to the body of Caroline Walsh and why were the anatomists at London Hospital apparently questioned not at all and their beadle only briefly? This last individual probably had the answers.

THE GARDNER MURDER

A few minutes before 8 A.M. on Monday, 15 September 1862, Mrs. Elizabeth Humbler knocked on the door of a surgeon, Henry Little Sequeira, to report in great distress that Mrs. Elizabeth Gardner had cut her throat. Sequeira and the woman hurried to the scene, a walk of about twenty minutes. Later, it developed that Mrs. Humbler, nineteen years old, lived with the Gardners and had recently been the husband's mistress. She and Samuel Gardner, the husband, were indicted for the murder. However, when the trial opened it was decided that there was no evidence against the Humbler girl. Her testimony being wanted, the jury on direction of the court at once acquitted her.

Henry Sequeira testified how he found Mrs. Gardner's body lying on the floor of a bedroom:

> I placed my hand first on the thing, and found that it was quite cold—part of the body was warm, just the lower part of the trunk; the upper part, the shoulders, was quite cold. . . . I thought she had been dead four hours. . . . The left hand was on the chest. . . . the right hand was also on the chest and held a knife . . . . I afterwards noticed that there was an impression, a sooty impression on the left elbow, and also on the left wrist, on the inside; it was plainly, as I mentioned to the Coroner, a digital impression, finger marks, sooty. . . . the throat was cut, and there was a pool of blood under both sides of the throat. . . . the wound on the throat was about two inches and a quarter in length, from the apple of the throat downwards to the shoulder on the left side. . . . I considered that it commenced from the front of the throat. . . . it was deepest externally near the shoulder.
>
> *Q.* In your judgment was it such a wound as the woman could have inflicted herself? *A.* She could not have done it with her right hand.

Two or three minutes after he and the Humbler woman hurried into the room, Sequeira continued, Samuel Gardner entered. He said, "What is this?" and immediately took the knife from the victim's hand.

> MR. POLAND. *Q.* Had he any difficulty in getting the knife from the hand? *A.* No difficulty at all—it left the hand as easily as it leaves mine—the back of the knife was against the palm of the deceased's hand, and it was in that position, so that the back of the knife was toward the throat . . . .
>
> MR. POLAND. *Q.* Supposing the woman had died with the knife in her hand, would the hand have been contracted? *A.* It would have been firmly clasped around the knife.

After Gardner picked up the weapon, he accused Elizabeth Humbler of the murder. She denied this.

> Q. Did you see any marks of any kind upon Humbler, any marks of blood upon her clothers? *A.* [Sequeira] I saw her hands examined by the policeman in my presence, and I did not see anything upon her hands except dirt—they did not appear to have been washed for some time.

Sequeira found defense cuts on the victim's hands as if she had laid hold of the knife, the direction "corresponding with that in the palm. . . . the insides of the hands appeared as if they had been wiped. . . . on the thigh there was an impress of the palm of a hand, and a thumb. . . . I could trace the mark of the thumb distinctly, it was pointing downwards; it was broader than my hand."

The surgeon was questioned again about the fatal neck wound. He was sure that "the wound was deepest at the further extremity—I say it is impossible that the wound could have been inflicted with the right hand . . . . the direction . . . was downwards, backwards and inwards towards the spinal column."

The same witness stated that he had made a post-mortem examination and found Mrs. Gardner to be seven months pregnant. A second surgeon confirmed Sequeira's observations and opinion, including the assertion that by 8 A.M. the victim had been dead for four or five hours.

Gardner, the accused, was a chimney sweep and began his labors early in the morning. He admitted that he had left his house at 4 A.M. on the morning of the attack. He also stated that "Deceased was not left-handed." On the day of the murder Gardner had been seen on the street by various witnesses at several times between 4:30 and 7 A.M.

A good deal of additional evidence was heard, the defense trying to make a case for suicide, but Sequeira's careful and astute observations, confirmed by his colleague, convinced the jury, and the chimney sweep was condemned to death (*OB,* Oct. 1862: pp. 708–33). The indication from body temperature that the attack must have occurred before Gardner left home, the admitted lack of evidence against the Humbler woman, including the absence of blood on her clothes and on her unwashed hands, the sooty handprint, the defense cuts, the nature and direction of the fatal wound, Gardner's admission that his wife was right-handed, and the position and loose grasp of the knife in the victim's hand, taken together, built a very strong case against the husband.

Sequeira had estimated the temperature of the body by simple palpation, a procedure, he added, which he had performed hundreds of times in the course of a large medical practice. As a result of the Gardner case, A. S. Taylor and Samuel Wilks in a unique investigation made temperature determinations on one hundred dead bodies at Guy's Hospital "by simply placing the bulb of a thermometer on the skin of the abdomen" (Taylor and Wilks, 1863). Following this work, other important observations on post-mortem changes in body temperature and on the factors responsible were published during the next decade. Woodman and Tidy add that Dr. Henry Letheby showed them manuscript notes of similar studies made by him as early as 1851 (Woodman and Tidy, 1877: p. 38ff.) but the Gardner murder seems to be the first homicide reported in the *Sessions Papers* in which a careful post-mortem estimate of the time of death was based on body temperature.

THE WAINWRIGHT MURDER

Henry Wainwright, aged thirty-seven, well-educated, popular, by all appearance an upright citizen, was a married man with five children. He had formerly owned a brush-making business. One September evening in 1875, he asked Alfred P. Stokes, once an employee, to carry a parcel for him. Stokes agreeing, they went to a building at 215 Whitechapel Road. On the second floor Wainwright dug out of a pile of straw two large parcels wrapped in black American cloth, a kind of oilcloth, and tied with rope. He also handed Stokes a shovel and chopper, asking him to sell them. Stokes complained about an evil-smelling smear on the chopper, which Wainwright then wiped off with a newspaper. The helper grumbled also about the parcels—"They stink so bad and the weight of them is too heavy for me." After peering out the front door, Wainwright ordered, "All right, Stokes, no one is looking, come on," and off they went down Whitechapel Road, the former brush manufacturer carrying one bundle and Stokes the other. In the light of later events, Wainwright's effrontery was remarkable.

Stokes complained again at the weight he was carrying and Wainwright went for a cab. In his absence, the unwilling and by now suspicious porter "looked at the largest parcel, the one I carried myself; I felt as if I must do it—I opened it, and the first thing I saw was a human head, and then proceeding further I saw a hand which had been cut off at the wrist, and then I had the presence of mind to *kiver* it up again quick and wait till Mr. Wainwright returned with a four-wheeled cab." They put the parcels in the vehicle and Wainwright climbed in after them, telling Stokes he would see him that evening. The porter heard his former employer direct the driver to the Commercial Road.

Stokes managed to follow. He saw the cab stop while Wainwright spoke to a young woman named Alice Day. Then, said Stokes:

> they both got into the cab—I was hiding in a doorway opposite—he said to the cabman, "Drive on as fast as you can over London Bridge to the Borough [of Southwark]." . . . I ran after the cab until I saw two constables by Leadenhall Street—I called their attention to the cab as I was then exhausted, but they laughed at me and said "Man, you must be mad"—I called to them to stop the cab . . . . I ran after it again; it went . . . over London Bridge and stopped outside the hop factory . . . . I saw Wainwright . . . . he got out and took out the lightest parcel and went towards the Hen and Chickens—I told two constables, Turner and Cox, No. 48 and 290; I said "For God's sake run after the man with the high hat with the parcels in his hand, there is something wrong," and Turner done it instantly—I then told Cox, and he went to the cab . . . . Cox spoke to Alice Day but I could not hear the words—I saw Turner follow Wainwright to the Hen and Chickens on the other side—shortly afterwards Wainwright returned and went to the cab to get the other parcel.

The Hen and Chickens was an unoccupied public house formerly owned by Thomas Wainwright, brother of Henry. Alice Day, a ballet girl at the Pavilion Theatre in Whitechapel Road, was the latter's lady friend.

Cox and Turner escorted Henry Wainwright back into the Hen and Chickens. When the package was opened and found to contain parts of a human body, the brush maker offered the policemen £200 if they would let him go. Instead, the parcel was collected from the cab, and Wainwright and Alice Day were taken to the police station. There the second package was also opened, disclosing more portions of a decomposed, lime-covered body. The couple was "charged with having in their possession a human body decomposed, supposed to be murdered," surely an unusual complaint even in an East End police station that must have seen almost everything. The Day woman was soon discharged.

Under the floor of the Whitechapel Road brush factory that had formerly belonged to Henry Wainwright the police found a grave showing signs of earlier occupancy and containing numerous lumps of chloride of lime. Nearby were a hammer and a new chopper and spade coated with the same substance. The ten body parts were partly desiccated and partly transformed into adipocere.[14] The face was unrecognizable. Nevertheless, the body was suspected to be that of Harriet Louisa Lane. Now Henry Wainwright was charged with murder and his brother with being an accessory after the fact.

Under the name of Percy King the murderer had lived secretly with Harriet Lane and had had two children by her. Financial problems made it difficult for him to support his second family, and this and his growing lack of interest in Harriet led to quarrels. After moving several times, she departed from her last lodging on 11 September 1874, allegedly traveling by cab to the Whitechapel Road address to keep an appointment with Henry. Harriet Lane was never seen alive again. When her friends inquired from Wainwright, he indicated that she had gone away with another man. It was on 11 September 1875, exactly a year later, that the brush maker moved the parcels from the building in the Whitechapel Road. The reason, it developed, was that the property was about to be sold.

Much labor was expended by the police in the search for witnesses and for physical evidence, and when the Wainwrights came to trial in November the prosecution was ready with a formidable case. The testimony of the expert witnesses revealed some useful advances in forensic medical reasoning.

The earth in the grave was put through a screen, resulting in the recovery of a piece of rope, a wedding ring and keeper ring, two jet buttons, a human tooth, a knee cap, and a piece of scalp with hair. Two earrings and more buttons were found in the ashes under a grate in the Whitechapel Road premises.

A post-mortem examination was made by Frederick George Larkin and Thomas Bond, surgeons. Larkin testified that the victim was slender and about five feet tall. One ear could be examined; it was pierced. A bullet was found in the cerebellum and another in the sphenoid bone at the base of the skull. Fractures and holes showed that the bullets had entered the right side of the head, above and behind the ear. The surgeon observantly noted also "a little mark on the skull internally, where the bullet seems to have struck and rebounded." Blood extravasated around the bullet holes and under the scalp indica-

14. A waxy, soaplike substance formed by the action on body fat of moisture, calcium and ammonium ions, and bacteria.

ted that the shooting had occurred before the circulation was stopped by death. A third bullet had not entered the head, having lodged in dense rolls of wool that were held in place by hairpins and ribbons under the woman's hair at the back of her head.

In addition, the throat had been forcefully cut from the right to left, from the larynx upward to near the left angle of the jaw. This injury, it was made clear, had not been inflicted at the time of dismemberment; extravasated blood around the throat wound indicated that "the cut must have been made either immediately before or immediately after death." Questioned as to the possibility of suicide, Bond testified that the fatal shooting precluded the possibility that she had deeply cut her throat, and vice versa. Larkin had already expressed a similar opinion. As the judge pointed out in his summing-up, to assume suicide would mean believing that the dead woman had dug her own grave.

Hair mixed with lime and clay was found on the new spade; "it was hair of a light colour—I have part of it here—I saw the hair that was on the body, and it seemed to me exactly the same colour." A woman friend also said this hair, light auburn, was the same color as Harriet Lane's hair. Thomas Bond compared hair from the spade "with some of the hair from the body with a microscope—they corresponded in colour and substance, and in the markings of the medullary substance—I was shown some hair by Inspector Fox—I examined that in the same way with a microscope, and that also corresponded with the hair from the body." Ashes from the grate were also studied under the microscope, apparently without useful result.

Harriet Lane's father gave her age as twenty-four years. Two women friends testified that the missing Harriet had one decayed tooth; "it was in the upper jaw, the one next to the eye tooth . . . . it showed when she laughed and talked." Larkin, the surgeon, gave it as his opinion that the victim "was about 25 years of age, from the condition of the wisdom teeth; all the wisdom teeth were cut except one, which was evidently being cut at the time.[15] . . . I noticed that one tooth was decayed down level with the gum or jaw; and only one, as far as I could see—it was the next tooth behind the eye tooth on the right side." The teeth, found separate from the body, corresponded to empty sockets in the jaws of the murdered woman.

15. Human third molar teeth usually erupt between the ages of seventeen and twenty-five (Hamilton, 1976: pp. 339).

It was estimated that Harriet Lane had been dead roughly from nine to twelve months. The criteria on which this opinion was based were not specified.

The dead woman was known to have had a scar the size of a shilling from a childhood burn. It was about four inches below her right knee on the outer side of the leg. Just such a scar was found on the victim's leg.

As already noted, Harriet Lane and Henry Wainwright had had two children, born in August 1872 and December 1873. At the post-mortem examination the uterus was carefully examined for signs of past pregnancy. Larkin expressed the opinion, based on measurements, that the victim had indeed born a child. He also observed that the lower abdominal skin of the dead woman showed the white lines or *lineae albicantes* which may appear during, and persist after, pregnancy.

Mr. Bond disagreed with his fellow surgeon, doubting that the uterus had ever been pregnant. Wisdom teeth, he said, "sometimes come late in life, sometimes over thirty years of age—I think it is impossible to fix the age of a person whose remains these were within ten years."

Dr. Alfred Meadows, a lecturer on midwifery at St. Mary's Hospital, examined the uterus but not the rest of the body. He found it "not possible to express any distinct opinion as to whether the uterus had been pregnant or not; my opinion, considering the points mentioned, is that the uterus had not been pregnant."

Frederick George Aubyn, surgeon, also doubted that pregnancy had occurred. Like some other witnesses, he detected slight differences in the color of hair samples but suggested that the chloride of lime could have had a bleaching effect. Aubyn thought the woman's age had been about twenty-five because the anterior and posterior sutures of the skull had not yet closed.

Flag stones near the grave in the warehouse showed cuts and indentations that could have been produced with the chopper. On 10 September a shop keeper had sold Henry Wainwright eight yards of rope similar to that found at the grave. An upholsterer on the same day had sold him two yards of black American cloth. Thomas Wainwright, ever the businessman, later told a policeman of buying a spade and wood chopper, also on 10 September, for his elder brother; "I paid 3*s*., and I charged my brother 5*s*." The ironmonger who made the sale explained that "I charged him [Thomas] 3*s*. for the two as he was in the trade; the real price would have been 5*s*." However, the ironmonger could not be certain that the spade and chopper exhibited in court had come from his shop. A milliner friend of Harriet Lane testified that the buttons exhibited in court resembled those with which the missing woman's dress had been trimmed. An unsuccessful attempt was made to relate the bullets removed from the body to a gun to which Wainwright might have had access.

After a trial lasting from 22 to 30 November, Henry Wainwright was found guilty. Still protesting his innocence, he was sentenced to death. Thomas Wainwright, the younger brother, was convicted as an accessory after the fact and was sentenced to seven years' penal servitude.[16] Detailed autopsy reports by Larkin and Bond, and Meadows's comments on the uterus, subsequently published in the *British Medical Journal*,[17] brought an end to the record of one of Britain's most sensational murder cases.

16. *OB,* Nov. 1875: pp. 3–90; Wainwright, 1875a, b; Woodman and Tidy, 1877: pp. 1048–49; Irving, 1920.

17. Bond, 1875; Larkin, 1875; Wainwright, 1875b.

APPENDIX

EARLY BOOKS IN ENGLISH ON FORENSIC MEDICINE

The following chronological list is, I believe, comprehensive up to 1878; a few volumes may have been overlooked. Because English forensic medicine was influenced by American works on the subject, significant early examples of the latter are included. Also listed are certain important published lectures and syllabi. Some of the books on psychiatry touch only peripherally on forensic medicine.

Only first editions have been noted; short titles have been used. The titles and editions that follow are not necessarily cited in the text of this book.

Farr, Samuel. 1788. *Elements of medical jurisprudence*. London: T. Becket.

Dease, William. 1792. *Remarks on medical jurisprudence*. Dublin: P. Byrne.

[Percival, Thomas. 1794.] *Medical jurisprudence*. Manchester: [no pub.].

Duncan, Andrew. 1795. *Heads of lectures on medical jurisprudence*. Edinburgh: [no pub.].

Johnstone, John. 1800. *On madness*. Birmingham: S. Belcher.

Rush, Benjamin. 1811. *Sixteen introductory lectures*. Philadelphia: Bradford & Innskeep.

Stringham, J. S. 1814. *American medical and philosophical register*. (Cited by Ackerknecht and Kozelka, 1950: p. 1306.)

Bartley, O. W. 1815. *Treatise on forensic medicine or medical jurisprudence*. Bristol: Barry.

Male, G. E. 1816. *An epitome of juridical or forensic medicine*. London: T. & G. Underwood.

Beck, J. B. 1817. *An inaugural dissertation on infanticide*. New York: J. Seymour.

Haslam, John. 1817. *Medical jurisprudence as it relates to insanity*. London: C. Hunter.

Cooper, Thomas. 1819. *Tracts on medical jurisprudence*. Philadelphia: James Webster.

Smith, J. G. 1821. *The principles of forensic medicine*. London: T. & G. Underwood.

Beck, T. R. 1823. *Elements of medical jurisprudence*. Albany: Webster & Skinner.

Paris, J. A., and J. S. M. Fonblanque. 1823. *Medical jurisprudence*. London: W. Phillips.

Smith, J. G. 1825. *An analysis of medical evidence*. London: T. & G. Underwood.

Christison, Robert. 1826. *Syllabus of the University course of lectures on medical jurisprudence*. Edinburgh: J. Balfour.

Dunglison, [Robley]. 1827. *Syllabus of the lectures on medical jurisprudence.* [Charlottesville, Va.]: University of Virginia: C. P. M'Kennie.
Christison, Robert. 1829. *A treatise on poisons.* Edinburgh: A. Black.
Forsyth, J. S. 1829. *A synopsis of modern medical jurisprudence.* London: W. Benning.
Conolly, John. 1830. *An inquiry concerning the indications of insanity.* London: John Taylor.
Willcock, J. H. 1830. *The laws relating to the medical profession.* London: A. Strahan.
Burrows, George. 1831. *Introductory lecture to a course on forensic medicine.* London: J. Mallett.
Ryan, Michael. 1831. *A manual of medical jurisprudence.* London: Renshaw and Rush.
Severn, Charles. 1831. *First lines of the practice of midwifery.* London: S. Highley. (Contains section on feticide and infanticide.)
Thomson, A. T. 1831. *Lecture introductory to the course of medical jurisprudence.* London: John Taylor.
Beck, J. B. 1835. *Researches in medicine and medical jurisprudence.* New York: E. Bliss.
Williams, S. W. 1835. *A catechism of medical jurisprudence.* Northampton, Mass.: J. H. Butler.
Chitty, J. 1836. *A practical treatise on medical jurisprudence.* Philadelphia: Carey, Lea & Blanshard. (Part 1; part 2 was never published.)
Cummin, William. 1836. *The proofs of infanticide considered.* London: Longman.
Taylor, A. S. 1836. *Elements of medical jurisprudence.* London: Deacon.
Traill, A. S. 1836. *Outlines of a course of lectures on medical jurisprudence.* Edinburgh: Black.
Watson, Alexander. 1837. *Medico-legal treatise on homicide by external violence.* Edinburgh: Maclachlan & Stewart.
Ray, [Isaac]. 1838. *A treatise on the medical jurisprudence of insanity.* Boston: Little & Brown.
Dean, Amos. 1840. *Manual of medical jurisprudence for the use of his class.* Albany: J. Munsell.
Pagan, J. M. 1840. *The medical jurisprudence of insanity.* London: Ball, Arnold.
Skae, David. [1840]. *Cases in legal medicine.* Edinburgh: J. Stark.
Sampson, M. B. 1841. *Criminal jurisprudence considered in relation to mental organization.* London: Samuel Highley.
Prichard, J. C. 1842. *On the different forms of insanity, in relation to jurisprudence.* London: Baillière.
Winslow, Forbes. 1843. *The plea of insanity in criminal cases.* London: H. Renshaw.
Guy, W. A. 1844. *Principles of forensic medicine.* London: H. Renshaw.
Taylor, A. S. 1844. *A manual of medical jurisprudence.* London: J. Churchill.
______. 1848. *On poisons in relation to medical jurisprudence and medicine.* London: J. Churchill.
Dean, Amos. 1850. *Principles of medical jurisprudence.* Albany: Gould, Banks & Gould.

Storer, D. H. 1851. *An address on medical jurisprudence.* Boston: John Wilson.
Wharton, Francis, and Moreton Stillé. 1855. *A treatise on medical jurisprudence.* Rochester, N.Y.: Lawyers' Cooperative.
Gilman, C. R. 1856. *The relations of the legal to the medical profession.* New York: Baker & Godwin.
Robinson, George. 1856. *Observations on some recent cases of poisoning.* Gateshead, Co. Durham: D. Dunglison.
Wynne, James. 1859. *Importance of the study of legal medicine.* New York and London: H. Baillière.
Elwell, J. J. 1860. *A medico-legal treatise on malpractice and medical evidence.* New York: J. S. Voorhies.
Casper, J. L. 1861–65. *A handbook of the practice of forensic medicine.* Trans. G. W. Balfour. London: New Sydenham Soc.
Ryan, W. B. 1862. *Infanticide: Its law, prevalence, prevention, and history.* London: J. Churchill.
Taylor, A. S. 1865. *The principles and practice of medical jurisprudence.* London: J. Churchill.
Wormley, T. G. 1867. *Micro-chemistry of poisons.* New York: H. Baillière.
Husband, H. A. 1874. *The students' handbook of forensic medicine and medical police.* Edinburgh: E. & S. Livingstone.
Woodman, W. B., and C. M. Tidy. 1877. *Forensic medicine and toxicology.* Philadelphia: Lindsay & Blakiston.
Ogston, Francis. 1878. *Lectures on medical jurisprudence.* Philadelphia: Lindsay & Blakiston.

REFERENCES

Ackerknecht, E. H., and F. L. Kozelka. 1950. Early history of legal medicine. *Ciba Symp.* 11:1286–1316.

Adelson, Lester. 1952. Spontaneous human combustion and preternatural combustibility. *J. Crim. Law, Criminology and Police Science.* 42:793–809.

———. 1974. *The pathology of homicide. . . .* Springfield, Ill.: Thomas.

Alderson, James. 1856. Deaths from poison. *Lancet.* 1 80.

Allderidge, P. A. 1974. Criminal insanity: Bethlem to Broadmoor. *Proc. Roy. Soc. Med.* 67:897–904.

Allnatt, R. H. 1836. Morison's pills: Another example of their deleterious nature. *London Med. Gaz.* 17:415–16.

Atkinson, S. B. 1904. Life, birth, and live-birth. *Quart. Law Rev.* 20:134–59.

Atlay, J. B., ed. 1911. *Trial of the Stauntons.* Edinburgh: Wm. Hodge.

Babington, Anthony. 1971. *The English Bastille. . . .* London: Macdonald.

Baillie, Matthew. 1793. *The morbid anatomy of some of the most important parts of the human body.* London: J. Johnson & G. Nicol.

Baker, J. H. 1971. *An introduction to English legal history.* London: Butterworths.

Baldwin [no initials]. 1819. An account of the Proceedings of the Society for Superseding the Necessity of Climbing Boys. *Edinburgh Rev.* 32:309–20.

Bannister, Roger. 1978. *Brain's Clinical neurology.* Oxford: Oxford University Press.

Bartholin, Thomas. 1663. *Bartholinus Anatomy. . . .* London: Peter Cole.

Bartley, O. W. 1815. *Treatise on forensic medicine or medical jurisprudence* Bristol: Barry & Son.

Bartsch, Karl. 1920. Chrestomathie de l'ancien Français (VIIIe–XVe siècles). . . . Leipzig: F. C. W. Vogel.

Battie, William. 1758. *A treatise on madness.* London: J. Whiston & B. White.

Beck, J. B. 1817. *An inaugural dissertation on infanticide. . . .* New York: J. Seymour.

———. 1835. *Researches in medicine and medical jurisprudence.* New York: E. Bliss.

———. [1842]. *Observations on some of the signs of live and still birth. . . .* [N.p.].

Beck, T. R. 1823. *Elements of medical jurisprudence.* Albany: Webster & Skinners.

———, and J. B. Beck. 1835. *Elements of medical jurisprudence.* Albany: Steele, Skinner, Little & Gould.

Beckett, William 1718, 1720. An attempt to prove the antiquity of the venereal disease. . . . *Phil. Trans. Roy. Soc. London,* 30:839–47; 31:47–65, 108–12.

Behlmer, G. K. 1979. Deadly motherhood: Infanticide and medical opinion in mid-Victorian England. *J. Hist. Med. Allied Sci.* 34:403–27.

Bell, John. 1848. *Syllabus of a course of lectures. . . .* Philadelphia: [no pub.].

Berridge, Virginia. 1979. Opium in the fens in nineteenth-century England. *J. Hist. Med. Allied Sci.* 34:293–313.

Bianchini, Francesco, and Francesco Corbetta. 1977. *Health plants of the world.* New York: Newsweek Books.

Biggs, John, Jr. 1955. *The guilty mind: Psychiatry and the law of homicide.* Baltimore: Johns Hopkins University Press.

Black, H. C. 1968. *Black's Law dictionary. . . .* St. Paul, Minn.: West.

Blackstone, William. 1872. *Commentaries. . . .* Chicago: Callaghan.

Bohn, Johannes. 1689. *De renunciatione vulnerum. . . .* Leipzig: J. F. Gleditsch.

———. 1690. *Specimen medicinae forensis.* Leipzig: Banckmann.

———. 1711. De infanticidio. In Johannes Bohn. *De renunciatione vulnerum,* pp. 169–92. Leipzig: Thomas Fritsch.

Bond, Thomas. 1875. The Whitechapel tragedy: Notes of a report to the Solicitor to the Treasury on the post mortem examination of remains. *Brit. Med. J.* 2:732.

Bonet, Théophile. 1679. *Sepulchretum, sive anatomia practica ex cadaveribus morbo denatis.* Geneva: L. Chouët.

Bray, R. A. 1911. *Boy labour and apprenticeship.* London: Constable.

Bremner, M. D. K. 1954. *The story of dentistry.* Brooklyn: Dental Items of Interest.

Brittain, R. P. 1963. The hydrostatic and similar tests of live birth: A historical review. *Med.-Leg. J.* 31:189–94.

———. 1965. Cruentation in legal medicine and in literature. *Med. Hist.* 9:82–88.

Brodie, B. C. 1811. Experiments and observations on the different modes in which death is produced by certain vegetable poisons. *Phil. Trans. Roy. Soc. London.* 101:178–208.

———. 1812. Further experiments and observations on the action of poisons on the animal system. Ibid. 102:205–27.

Brodrick, Norman. 1971. *Report of the Committee on Death Certification and Coroners. . . .* London: H. M. Stationery Office.

Browne, D. G., and E. V. Tullett. 1951. *Bernard Spilsbury: His life and cases.* London: G. C. Harrap.

Browne, G. L., and C. G. Stewart. 1883. *Reports of trials for murder by poisoning. . . .* London: Stevens.

Burnett, John. 1811. *A treatise on various branches of the criminal law of Scotland.* Edinburgh: George Ramsay.

Burnett, John. 1969. *A history of the cost of living.* Harmondsworth, Middlesex: Penguin.

Burrows, George. 1831. *Introductory lecture to a course on forensic medicine. . . .* London: J. Mallett.

1953. *Calendar of the close rolls. . . .* London: H. M. Stationery Office.

Campbell, W. A. 1965. Some landmarks in the history of arsenic testing. *Chem. in Britain.* 1:198–202.

———. 1981. The history of the chemical detection of poisons. *Med. Hist.* 25:202–03.

Camps, F. E., ed. 1968. The history of legal medicine. In *Gradwohl's legal medicine.* Baltimore: Williams & Wilkins.

Carter, A. T. 1910. *A history of English legal institutions.* London: Butterworths.

Castro, Rodrigo de. 1614. *Medicus-politicus. . . .* Hamburg: Froben.

1876. Central Criminal Court, 31 May, 1 June. *London Times,* 1, 2 June.

Chaillé, S. E. 1876. Origin and progress of medical jurisprudence, 1776–1876. *Trans. Internat. Med. Cong. Phila.* [n. pp.]. Reprinted in 1949. *J. Crim. Law Criminol.* 40:397–444.

Chapman, C. B. 1982. Stratton vs. Swanlond: The fourteenth-century ancestor of the law of malpractice. *Pharos.* 45:20–24.

1838. Charing Cross Hospital Medical School. *Minute Book of School Committee of Management.* MS. 6 July.

Chevallier, A. 1834. Rapports judiciaires faits dans le but de reconnaître la nature de taches sur le linge. *Ann. D'Hyg. publ. et Méd. leg.* 11:210–23.

Chitty, J. 1836. *A practical treatise on medical jurisprudence. . . .* Part 1. Philadelphia: Carey, Lea & Blanchard.

Christison, Robert. 1826. *Syllabus of the University course of lectures on medical jurisprudence. Edinburgh: A. Balfour.*

———. 1829a. *A treatise on poisons.* Edinburgh: A. Black.

———. 1829b. Case IV. Murder by suffocation. Injury of the spine after death imitating an injury during life.—Experiments on the effects of blows soon after death. *Edinb. Med. Surg. J.* 31:236–50. Reprinted in 1972. *Forensic Sci.* 1:119–31.

———. 1829c. Cases and observations in medical jurisprudence.—III. Disfiguring of the countenance with sulphuric acid.—IV. Murder by suffocation. . . . *Edinb. Med. Surg. J.* 31:229–50.

———. 1845. *A treatise on poisons.* . . . Philadelphia: Ed. Barrington & Geo. D. Haswell.

City of London sessions minutes for 1691/92. Gaol delivery for 24 February. MS. SM62: Corporation of London Record Office.

Clarke, James. 1808. Report from "the General Hospital near Nottingham." *Edinb. Med. Surg. J.* 4:265–85.

Clarke, Karen. 1980. Infanticide, illegitimacy and the medical profession in nineteenth century England. *Soc. Social Hist. Med. Bull.* No. 26:11–14.

Coke, Edward. 1794. *First part of the institutes of the laws of England.* . . . London: E. & R. Brooke. *1*, bk. 3, chap. 6, sect. 405.

1971. *The compact edition of the Oxford English dictionary.* Oxford: Oxford University Press.

Condronchi, Baptista. 1597. *De vitiis vocis, libri duo. . . . Cui accedit . . . methodus testificandi.* . . . Frankfurt: A. Wechel.

Conolly, John. 1830. *An inquiry concerning the indications of insanity.* . . . London: John Taylor. Reprinted with introduction by Richard Hunter and Ida Macalpine. 1964. London: Dawson's.

Cooper, Samuel. 1830. *The first lines of the practice of surgery.* Philadelphia: J. Grigg.

Cooper, Thomas. 1819. *Tracts on medical jurisprudence.* . . . Philadelphia: James Webster.

Cornelius, E. H. 1978. John Hunter as an expert witness. *Ann. Roy. Coll. Surg. England.* 60:412–18.

Cosman, M. P. 1972. Medieval medical malpractice and Chaucer's physician. *N.Y. State Med. J.* 72:2439–44.

———. 1973. Medieval medical malpractice: The dicta and the dockets. *Bull. N.Y. Acad. Med.* 49:22–47.

Creighton, Charles. 1965. *A history of epidemics in Britain.* London: Frank Cass.

Cummin, W. 1833. Practice of forensic medicine, as conducted in this and other countries. *London Med. Gaz.* 13:951–52.

———. 1836. *The proofs of infanticide considered.* . . . London: Longman.

Cumston, C. G. 1910. Remarks on the history of forensic medicine from the renaissance to the XIX century. *Med. Record.* Oct.: 1–15.

———. 1912–13. A note on the history of forensic medicine of the Middle Ages. *J. Amer. Inst. Criminol.* 3:855–65.

1938. *Curia regis rolls of the reign of Henry III.* . . . London: H. M. Stationery Office.

Curran, W. J. 1975. The confusion of titles in the medicolegal field: An historical analysis and a proposal for reform. *Med. Sci. Law.* 15:270–75.

Damme, Catherine. 1978. Infanticide: The worth of an infant under law. *Med. History.* 22:1–24.

Davies, D. S. 1937. Child-killing in English law. *Modern Law Rev.* 1:203–23, 269–87.

Davis, B. T. 1973. George Edward Male MD—the father of English medical jurisprudence. *Proc. Roy. Soc. Med.* 67:117–20.

Davison, M. H. A. 1964. Medicine, murder, and man. *Med.-Legal J.* 32:28–39.

Dean, Amos. 1840. *Manual of medical jurisprudence for the use of his class.* Albany: J. Munsell.

———. 1854. *Principles of medical jurisprudence.* Albany: Gould, Banks.

Deans, R. S. 1921. *The students' legal history.* London: Stevens.

Dease, William. 1792. *Remarks on medical jurisprudence.* . . . Dublin: P. Byrne.

———. 1819. Remarks on medical jurisprudence. . . . In Thomas Cooper. *Tracts on medical jurisprudence.* Philadelphia: James Webster.

1836. Death from quack medicine: Morison's pills. *London Med. Gaz.* 17:357–58.

DeFord, M. A. 1960. *The Overbury affair. . . .* Philadelphia: Chilton.
Dickens, Charles. 1906. *A tale of two cities.* New York: Macmillan.
1862. Diseased meat as human food. *Lancet.* 2:542.
1865. Diseased meat. *Lancet.* 2:635.
Dobson, Jessie. 1969. *John Hunter.* Edinburgh: E. & S. Livingstone.
1831. Domestic occurrences. *Gentleman's Mag.* 101 [Nov.]: 461, 643.
Donley, J. E. 1909. John James Wepfer, a Renaissance student of apoplexy. *Bull. Johns Hopkins Hosp.* 20:1–23.
Douglas, Hugh. 1973. *Burke and Hare: The true story.* London: Robert Hale.
Drayton, Michael. 1932. *Works.* Oxford: Blackwell.
Dreher, R. H. 1967. Origin, development, and present studies of insanity as a defense to criminal responsibility in common law. *J. History Behavioral Sci.* 3:47–57.
Dreisbach, R. H. 1980. *Handbook of poisoning. . . .* Los Altos, Calif: Lange.
Duncan, Andrew. 1795. *Heads of lectures on medical jurisprudence. . . .* Edinburgh: [no pub.].
———. 1807. A short view of the extent and importance of medical jurisprudence, considered as a branch of education. *Dublin Med. Phys. Essays.* 1:238–43.
Dunglison, [Robley]. 1827. *Syllabus of the lectures on medical jurisprudence. . . .* University of Virginia: C. P. M'Kennie.
———. 1868. *A dictionary of medical science. . . .* Philadelphia: H. C. Lea.
Earles, M. P. 1969. Introduction of chloral hydrate into medicine. *Pharmaceut. J.* 202:457–59.
Elwell, J. J. 1860. *A medico-legal treatise on malpractice and medical evidence. . . .* New York: J. S. Voorhies.
1692. The examination and confession of Edw. Francis blackamore servt. to Mr. Tho. Dymock. . . . *London General Sessions Papers,* Corporation of London Record Office. MS. 16 Jan.
Farr, Samuel. 1788. *Elements of medical jurisprudence. . . .* London: T. Becket.
———. 1819. Elements of medical jurisprudence. . . . In Thomas Cooper. *Tracts on medical jurisprudence.* Philadelphia: James Walker.
Farr, William. 1839. Letter to the Registrar-General. In *First annual report of the Registrar-General of births, deaths, and marriages in England.* London: W. Clowes.
———. 1840. Letter to the Registrar-General from William Farr, Esq. In *Second annual report of the Registrar-General of births, deaths, and marriages in England.* London: W. Clowes.
———. 1885. *Vital statistics. . . .* London: Edward Stanford.
Faselius, J. F. 1767. *Elementa medicinae forensis. . . .* Jena: J. W. Hartung.
Ficarra, B. J. 1977. History of legal medicine. *Legal Med. Ann.* 1976:3–27.
Fideli, Fortunato. 1602. *De relationibus medicorum. . . .* Palermo: I. A. de Francisco.
Flower, C. T., ed. 1944. Introduction to the curia regis rolls, 1199–1230 A.D. Selden Soc. 62. London: Quaritch.
Fodéré, F. E. 1798. *Les lois éclairées par les sciences physiques, ou Traité de médecine légale et d'hygiène publique.* Paris: Croullebois.
———. 1813. *Traité de medecine légale. . . .* Paris: de Mame.
Forbes, T. R. 1971. *Chronicle from Aldgate. . . .* New Haven: Yale University Press.
———. 1975. Percivall Pott performs a postmortem. *Bull. N.Y. Acad. Med.* 2nd ser., 51:272–76.
———. 1976a. Death of a chairman: A new William Hunter manuscript. *Yale J. Biol. Med.* 49:169–74.
———. 1976b. Malpractice and manslaughter: The case of Edward Martin Van Butchell. *Conn. Med.* 40:323–25.
———. 1977a. Inquests into London and Middlesex homicides, 1673–1782. *Yale J. Biol. Med.* 50:207–20.

______. 1977b. Coroners' inquests in the County of Middlesex, England, 1819–1842. *J. Hist. Med. Allied Sci. 32*:375–94.
______. 1978. Crowner's quest. *Trans. Amer. Philos. Soc.* 68:1–52.
______. 1980. John Hunter as expert witness. *Trans. Stud. Coll. Phys. Phila.* 5th ser. 2:75–80.
______. 1981a. A study of Old Bailey sentences between 1729 and 1800. *Guildhall Stud. Lond. Hist.* 5:26–35.
______. 1981b. Early forensic medicine in England: The Angus murder trial. *J. Hist. Med. Allied Sci.* 36:296–309.
Forsyth, J. S. 1829. *A synopsis of modern medical jurisprudence. . . .* London: W. Benning.
Foucault, Michel. 1978. About the concept of the "dangerous individual" in 19th century legal psychiatry. Trans. Alain Baudot and Jane Couchman. *Internat. J. Law Psychiatry.* 1:1–18.
Friedreich, J. B. 1844. Geschichtliches über den Ursprung der Lungenschwimmprobe. *Centralarch. f.d. ges. Staatsarzneikunde.* 1:337–45.
Garrison, F. H. 1929. *An introduction to the history of medicine. . . .* Philadelphia: Saunders.
1894. *General index to Guy's Hospital reports. Vols. I–L. 1836–1893.*
1777. *Gentleman's Mag.* 47:608.
1831a. Ibid. 101:461, 643.
1831b. Ibid. 101:553–54.
George, M. D. 1965. *London life in the 18th century.* New York: Capricorn.
Gettler, A. O. 1956. The historical development of toxicology, with interesting cases from the files of the Chief Medical Examiner's Office of New York City. *J. Forensic Sci.* 1:3–25.
Glaister, John. 1897. The history of medical jurisprudence and criminal procedure in primitive and mediaeval times. *Med. Times Hosp. Gaz.* 25:286–88, 302–04, 317–19.
______. 1928a. Forensic Medicine Department, University of Glasgow. In *Institutes of Legal Medicine.* 9th ser. New York: Division of Medical Education, Rockefeller Foundation.
______. 1928b. The evolution, development, and application of modern medico-legal methods. *Glasgow Med. J.* 109:417–37.
______. 1954. *The power of poison.* London: Christopher Johnson.
______. 1956. The trial of William Palmer. *St. Barth. Hosp. J.* 60:273–81.
______. 1960. The poisoner: Some aspects of famous trials. *Surgo* [*Glasgow Univ. Med. J.*] 26:82–88.
Gonzales, T. A., Morgan Vance, and Milton Helpern. 1937. *Legal medicine and toxicology.* New York: D. Appleton–Century.
Gorman, Mel. 1984. Sir William Brooke O'Shaughnessy, F. R. S. (1809–1889), Anglo-Indian forensic chemist. *Notes and Records Roy. Soc. London.* 39:51–64.
Greenfield, J. G. 1958. Traumatic lesions of the central and peripheral nervous systems. In J. G. Greenfield et al. *Neuropathology.* London: Edward Arnold.
Greenfield, W. S. 1877. Some remarks on the medical evidence in the Staunton case. *Lancet.* 2:492–95.
Greenwald, G. I., and M. W. Greenwald. 1981. Medicolegal progress in inquests of felonious deaths, Westminster, 1761–1866. *J. Legal Med.* 2:193–264.
Grimston, Harebotle. 1683a. *The first part of the reports of Sir George Croke, Kt. . . .* London: W. Rawlins, S. Roycroft, & H. Sawbridge.
______. 1683b. *The second part of the reports of Sir George Croke, Kt. . . .* London: W. Rawlins, S. Roycroft, & H. Sawbridge.
1963. *Guide to the contents of the Public Record Office.* London: H. M. Stationery Office.

Gurney, Joseph. 1817. *Brachygraphy, or short-hand made easy*. London: W. B. Gurney.
Guttmacher, A. F. 1935. Bootlegging bodies: A history of body-snatching. *Bull. Soc. Med. Hist. Chicago*. 4:353–402.
Guy, W. A. 1845. *Principles of forensic medicine*. New York: Harper.
Hale, Matthew. 1736. *Historia placitorum coronae*. . . . London: E. & R. Nutt & R. Gosling.
Haller, A. von. 1721. *Primae lineae physiologiae*. . . . Lausanne: Franc. Grasset.
Hamilton, W. A., ed. 1976. *Textbook of human anatomy*. St. Louis: Mosby.
Hand, Learned. 1901. Historical and practical considerations regarding expert testimony. *Harvard Law Rev*. 15:40–58.
Hansen, E. de G. R. 1979. "Overlaying" in 19th century England: Infant mortality or infanticide? *Human Ecol*. 7:333–52.
Harding, Alan. 1966. *A social history of English law*. Baltimore: Penguin.
Harvey, William. 1653. *Anatomical exercitations*. . . . London: James Young.
Haslam, John. 1819. *Medical jurisprudence as it relates to insanity*. . . . Philadelphia: James Webster.
Hatrick, W. R. 1862. Notes of twenty cases of poisoning. *Glasgow Med. J*. 10:381–402.
Havard, J. D. J. 1960. *The detection of secret homicide*. . . . London: Macmillan.
———. 1981. Medical jurisprudence. In *Encyclopaedia Britannica*. Chicago: Encyclopaedia Britannica.
Heddy, W. R. H. 1952. Some historic inquests. *Med.-Leg. J*. 20:122–30.
Helfand, W. H. 1974. James Morison and his pills. *Trans. Brit. Soc. Hist. Pharm*. 1:101–35.
Herman, J. R. 1978. Syphilis and gonorrhea are one disease: John Hunter (1760). *Internat. J. Dermatol*. 17:252–55.
1725. The history of the tryal of Richard Hunne, a citizen of London, for heresy after his death, and of Dr. Horsey, and others for murdering him, in the year 1514. In *The history of the most remarkable tryals in Great Britain and Ireland*. . . . London: J. Pemberton.
Hoffer, P. C., and N. E. H. Hull. 1981. *Murdering mothers*. . . . New York: New York University Press.
Holdsworth, William. 1966. *A history of English law*. London: Methuen.
Hovorka, O. von, and A. Kronfeld. 1909. *Vergleichende Volksmedizin*. Stuttgart: Strecker & Schröder.
Howarth, O. J. R. 1937. London. In *Encyclopaedia Britannica*. London: Encyclopaedia Britannica.
Howell, T. B. 1816. *A complete collection of state trials*. . . . London: Longman.
Howells, J. G., and M. L. Osborn. 1975. Great Britain. In J. G. Howells, ed. *World history of psychiatry*. New York: Brunner/Mazel.
Hunter, John. 1778. *The natural history of the human teeth*. London: J. Johnson.
———. 1794. *A treatise on the blood, inflammation, and gun-shot wounds*. London: G. Nicol.
———. 1837. On digestion of the stomach after death. In *Observations*. . . . London: Longman.
———. 1839. *Lectures on the principles of surgery*. Philadelphia: Haswell, Barrington, & Haswell.
Hunter, R. A., and Ida Macalpine. 1961. Dickens and Conolly: An embarrassed editor's disclaimer. *Times Lit. Suppl*. 11 Aug.:534–35.
———. 1962. *A treatise on madness by William Battie, M.D., and Remarks on Dr. Battie's Treatise on madness by John Monro, M.D. A psychiatric controversy of the eighteenth century*. London: Dawson's.

———. 1963. *Three hundred years of psychiatry, 1535–1860. . . .* London: Oxford University Press.
Hunter, William. 1783. On the uncertainty of the signs of murder, in the case of bastard children. *Med. Observ. Inqu.* 6:266–90.
Hunter, William. 1914. *Historical account of Charing Cross Hospital and Medical School (University of London). . . .* London: John Murray.
Hutchins, B. L., and A. Harrison. 1926. *A history of factory legislation.* London: P. S. King.
Hutchinson, W. 1820. On feticide. *London Med. Phys. J.* 43:90–98.
1847. Inhalation of ether. *London Med. Gaz.* N.s., 4:156–57.
1760. Inquest on William Robertson. *Greater London Records Office (Middlesex Records):* Accession 1268, Westminster Deps., MS. 21 May.
1855. Inquests and medical trials: Infants found dead in bed. *Lancet.* 1:103.
Irving, H. B., ed. 1920. *Trial of the Wainwrights.* Edinburgh: Wm. Hodge.
Jackson, A. D. M. 1982. "Wednesday's children": A review of child abuse. *J. Roy. Soc. Med.* 75:83–88.
1840. James Morison, Esq. *Gentleman's Mag.* 2:437–38.
James the First. 1597. *Daemonologie.* Reprinted 1924. London: John Lane.
Jenks, Edward. [1912]. *A short history of English law from the earliest times to the end of the year 1927.* London: Methuen.
Johnstone, John. 1800. *On madness.* Birmingham: S. Belcher.
Jones, Kathleen. 1955. *Lunacy, law and conscience, 1744–1845.* London: Routledge & Kegan Paul.
Jorden, Edward. 1603. *A briefe discourse of a disease called the suffocation of the mother. . . .* London: Windet.
Keele, K. D. 1965. *William Harvey: The man, the physician, and the scientist.* London: Nelson.
King, L. S., and M. C. Meehan. A history of the autopsy. *Amer. J. Path.* 73:514–44.
Knapp, Andrew, and William Baldwin. [1820?] *The new Newgate calendar.* Vols. 1, 2, London: J. Robins; vols. 3–5, London: J. & J. Cundee.
Knott, G. H., and E. R. Watson, eds. 1923. *Trial of William Palmer.* Edinburgh: Wm. Hodge.
Kölliker, R. A. von. 1852. *Handbuch der Gewebelehre des Menschen.* Leipzig: W. Engelmann.
Kramer, J. C. 1979. Opium rampant: Medical use, misuse and abuse in Britain and the West in the 17th and 18th centuries. *Brit. J. Addiction.* 74:377–89.
Kühn, C. G. 1822. *Medicorum graecorum opera.* Leipzig, C. Cnobloch.
Lambarde, William. 1602. *Eirenarcha, or of the Office of the justices of peace. . . .* London: Thomas Wight.
1877. *Lancet.* 2:502–03.
Langer, W. L. 1972. Checks on population growth: 1750–1850. *Scient. Amer.* 226:93–99.
———. 1974. Infanticide: A historical survey. *History Childhood.* 1:353–66.
Larkin, F. G. 1875. The Whitechapel tragedy: Report of the post mortem examination of the remains. *Brit. Med. J.* 2:730–31.
Lee, Sidney, ed. 1909. *Dictionary of national biography.* New York: Macmillan.
Lewinstein, S. R. 1969. The historical development of insanity as a defense in criminal actions. *J. Forensic Sci.* 14:275–93, 469–500.
Linebaugh, P. 1977. The Ordinary of Newgate and his *Account.* In J. S. Cockburn, ed. *Crime in England, 1550–1800.* Princeton, N.J.: Princeton University Press.
Littlejohn, Harvey. 1915. The teaching of forensic medicine. *Trans. Med.-Leg. Soc. (London).* 12:1–12.

Littlejohn, H. H. 1928. Department of Forensic Medicine, University of Edinburgh. In *Institutes of legal medicine*. New York: Division of Medical Education, Rockefeller Foundation.

Lodge, F. T. 1901. A half-century's progress in medical jurisprudence. *Phys. and Surg.* 23:49–59.

Lomax, Elizabeth. 1973. The uses and abuses of opiates in nineteenth-century England. *Bull. Hist. Med.* 47:167–76.

Long, E. R. 1928. *A history of pathology*. Baltimore: Williams & Wilkins.

Longmate, Norman. 1974. *The workhouse*. London: Temple Smith.

Louis, Antoine. 1764. *Mémoire contre la légitimité des naissances prétendues tardives*. Paris: P. G. Cavelier.

Macalpine, Ida, and Richard Hunter. [c. 1969]. *George III and the mad-business*. [London]: A. Lane.

Maitland, F. W., ed. 1887. *Bracton's note book*. . . . London: C. J. Clay.

Malcolmson, R. W. 1977. Infanticide in the eighteenth century. In J. S. Cockburn, ed. *Crime in England, 1550–1800*. Princeton, N.J.: Princeton University Press.

Male, G. E. 1816. *An epitome of juridical or forensic medicine*. . . . London: T. & G. Underwood.

______. 1819. An epitome of juridical or forensic medicine . . . . In Thomas Cooper, ed. *Tracts on medical jurisprudence*. . . . Philadelphia: James Webster.

Manchester, A. H. 1980. *A modern legal history of England and Wales, 1750–1950*. London: Butterworths.

Mant, A. K. 1971. Official medico-legal investigation under the coroner's system in London, England. *Med.-Leg. Bull.* 20:1–8.

______. Milestones in the development of the British medicolegal system. *Med., Sci., Law*. 17:155–63.

March, James. 1836. Account of a method of separating small quantities of arsenic from substances with which it may be mixed. *Edinb. New Philosoph. J.* 21:229–36.

Marshall, John. 1815. *Five cases of recovery from the effects of arsenic*. . . . London: C. Chapple.

______. 1817. *Remarks on arsenic*. . . . London: Callow.

Martin, P. J. 1826. Observations on some of the accidents of infanticide. *Edinb. Med. Surg. J.* 25:34–36.

Mason, A. H. B. 1980. Crime and anaesthesia-robbery. *Hist. Med.* 8:18–19, 32.

McElwee, William. 1952. *The murder of Sir Thomas Overbury*. New York: Oxford University Press.

McMenemey, W. H. 1968. Cellular pathology, with special reference to the influence of Virchow's teachings on medical thought and practice. In F. N. L. Poynter. *Medicine and science in the 1860's*. London: Wellcome Institute of the History of Medicine.

Mead, Richard. 1702. *A mechanical account of poisons in several essays*. London: J. R. for R. South.

1836. Medical jurisprudence. *Provincial Med. Surg. J.* 1:463–66.

1844. Medical jurisprudence. Ibid. 8:574–76.

1862. Memoir of Thomas Wakley, Esq. *Lancet*. 1:609–12.

Mettler, C. C. 1947. *History of medicine*. Philadelphia: Blakiston.

Monckton, D. H. 1856. The Rugeley suspected secret poisoning cases: Minutes of the post-mortem examinations of the bodies of Walter and Ann Palmer. *Lancet*. 1:188–91.

Monro, John. 1758. *Remarks on Dr. Battie's Treatise on madness*. London: John Clarke.

1861. More food for disease. *Lancet*. 1:144.

Morgagni, G. B. 1761. *De sedibus et causis morborum*. . . . Venice: Remondini.

———. 1763. *Opuscula miscellanea.* . . . Naples: D. Torres. Trans. W. H. Hewitt. 1972. *Forensic Sci.* 1:339–87.
———. 1769. *The seats and causes of diseases.* . . . Trans. Benjamin Alexander. London: A. Millar & T. Cadell.
Morgan, John, and Thomas Addison. 1829. *An essay on the operation of poisonous agents upon the living body.* London: Longman, Rees.
1834. "Morison's pills."—Charge of manslaughter. *Annual Register.* 76:305–09.
1836a. Morison's pills: Trial for manslaughter. *London Med. Gaz.* 18:74–78.
1836b. Morison's pills. Ibid. 17:623–24.
1836c. Morison's pills: Another verdict of manslaughter. Ibid. 17:832.
Mullinger, J. B. 1908. Fisher, John (1459–1535). In Leslie Stephen and Sidney Lee, eds. *Dictionary of national biography.* London: Macmillan.
Munk, William. 1878. *The roll of the Royal College of Physicians of London.* . . . London: The College.
Myers, R. O. 1962. Famous forensic scientists.—Alfred Swaine Taylor (1806–1880). *Med. Sci. Law.* 2:233–40.
Nagle, R. 1970. "A singular case" and Dr. Smethurst. *Med.-Leg. J.* 38:51–53.
Nemec, Jaroslav. [1973]. *International bibliography of the history of legal medicine.* Bethesda, Md.: U.S. Department of Health, Education and Welfare.
———. 1976. *Highlights in medicolegal relations.* Bethesda, Md.: U.S. Department of Health, Education and Welfare.
1858. *Nineteenth annual report of the Registrar-General.* . . . London: Eyre and Spottiswood.
Odgers, W. B. 1901. Changes in procedure and in the law of evidence. In *A century of law reforms.* . . . London: Macmillan.
Ogston, Francis. 1878. *Lectures on medical jurisprudence.* Philadelphia: Lindsay & Blakiston.
1942. Old Bailey. In *Encylopaedia Americana.* New York: Americana.
O'Neill, Y. V. 1976. Innocent III and the evolution of anatomy. *Med. Hist.* 20:429–33.
Ormrod, Roger. 1977. The McNaughton case and its predecessors. In D. J. West and Alexander Walk. *Daniel McNaughton: His trial and the aftermath.* [Ashford, Kent]: Gaskell.
Paine, W. W. 1937. Police. In *Encyclopaedia Britannica.* London: Encyclopaedia Britannica.
Paré, Ambroise. 1575. *Les oeuvres.* . . . Paris: Gabriel Buon.
Parey, Ambrose. 1634. *The works.* . . . Trans. Th. Johnson. London: Th. Cotes & R. Young.
Paris, J. A. and J. S. M. Fonblanque. 1823. *Medical jurisprudence.* London: W. Phillips.
Parker, Brian. 1973. The beginnings of toxicology. In Robert Christison. *A treatise on poisons.* New York: AMS Press.
Parry, E. A. 1925. *The Overbury mystery.* . . . London: Unwin.
Parry, L. A., ed. 1931. *Trial of Dr. Smethurst.* Edinburgh: Wm. Hodge.
———. 1932. *Criminal abortion.* London: John Bale, Sons & Danielsson.
Parry-Jones, W. L. 1973. English private madhouses in the eighteenth and nineteenth centuries. *Proc. Roy. Soc. Med.* 66:659–64.
Payne, G. H. 1916. *The child in human progress.* New York: G. P. Putnam.
[Percival, Thomas. 1794]. *Medical jurisprudence.* . . . Manchester: [no pub.].
Peters, Dolores. 1981. The British medical response to opiate addiction in the nineteenth century. *J. Hist. Med. Allied Sci.* 36:455–88.
Peterson, W. S. 1973. A tree under the organic or doctor's system and tree under the Hygeian or Morisonian system. Ibid. 28:166–67.
[Pettigrew]. 1818. Forensic medicine, in the case of Abraham Kesler, of Montgomery County, New-York. *Med. Repository.* 19:314–19.

Pickering, Danby. 1763. *The statutes at large. . . .* Cambridge: Joseph Bentham.

Pike, L. O. 1876. *A history of crime in England. . . .* London: Smith, Elder.

Pilling, H. H. 1970. Social change and the coronership. *Med. Sci. Law.* 10:238–43.

Ploucquet, W. G. 1786. *Commentarius medicus. . . .* Strasburg: A. Koenig.

Plucknett, T. F. T. 1956. *A concise history of the common law.* Boston: Little, Brown.

Poland, H. B. 1901. Changes in criminal law and procedure since 1800. In *A century of law reform. . . .* London: Macmillan.

Polson, C. J., and D. J. Gee. 1973. *The essentials of forensic medicine.* Oxford: Pergamon.

Pott, P[ercivall]. 1773. *Observations on the nature and consequences of those injuries to which the head is liable from external injuries.* London: Hawes, Clarke, & Collins.

Power, D'Arcy. 1930. *Plarr's Lives of the Fellows of the Royal College of Surgeons of England.* Bristol: John Wright.

Prichard, J. C. 1835. *A treatise on insanity and other disorders affecting the mind.* London: Sherwood, Gilbert, & Piper.

———. 1842. *On the different forms of insanity, in relation to jurisprudence. . . .* London: Baillière.

Quen, J. M. 1968. An historical view of the M'Naghten trial. *Bull. Hist. Med.* 42:43–51.

———. 1969. James Hadfield and medical jurisprudence of insanity. *N.Y. State J. Med.* 69:1221–26.

———. 1974. Anglo-American criminal insanity: An historical perspective. *J. Hist. Behavioral Sci.* 10:313–23.

Radbill, S. X. 1968. A history of child abuse and infanticide. In R. E. Helfer and C. H. Kempe, eds. *The battered child.* Chicago: University of Chicago Press.

———. 1974. Pediatrics. In A. G. Debus, ed. *Medicine in the seventeenth century.* Berkeley: University of California Press.

Raithby, John. 1823. *Statutes. . . .* London: George Eyre & Andrew Strahan.

Ray, I[saac]. 1838. *A treatise on the medical jurisprudence of insanity.* Boston: Little & Brown.

Rayger, Karel. 1675–76. Miscellanea curiosa medicophysica. Cited by Jaroslav Nemec. 1976. *Highlights in medicolegal relations.* Bethesda, Md.: U.S. Department of Health, Education and Welfare.

Reid, John. 1841. Contributions to forensic medicine. *London & Edinb. Monthly J. Med. Sci.* 1:17–23.

Rembar, Charles. 1980. *The law of the land. . . .* New York: Simon & Schuster.

Rentoul, Edgar, and Hamilton Smith, eds. 1973. *Glaister's Medical jurisprudence and toxicology.* Edinburgh: Churchill Livingstone.

1817a. Review of: John Marshall. Remarks on arsenic. . . . London: Callow. 1817. *London Med. Repository.* 8:149–63.

1817b. Review of: John Marshall. Remarks on arsenic. . . . London, 1817. *Edinb. Med. Surg. J.* 13:507–20.

Rickards, G. K. 1861. *Statutes. . . .* London: Eyre & Spottiswoode.

Riley, H. T. 1868. *Memorials of London and London life in the XIIIth, XIVth, and XVth centuries. . . .* London: Longmans, Green.

Robinson, George. 1856. *Observations on some recent cases of poisoning.* Gateshead, Co. Durham: D. Dunglinson.

Rodin, A. E. 1973. *The influence of Matthew Baillie's Morbid anatomy. . . .* Springfield, Ill.: C C Thomas.

Rogers, H. W. 1891. *The law of expert testimony.* St. Louis: Central Law Journal Co.

Rosen, George. 1958. *A history of public health.* New York: MD Publicns.

Rosenberg, Albert. 1957. The Sarah Stout murder case: An early example of the doctor as an expert witness. *J. Hist. Med. Allied Sci.* 12:61–70.

Roughead, William, ed. 1914. *Trial of Mary Blandy*. Edinburgh: Wm. Hodge.
Rumbelow, Donald. 1971. *I spy blue. . . .* London: Macmillan.
Rush, Benjamin. 1811. *Sixteen introductory lectures*. Philadelphia: Bradford & Inns-keep. Reprinted with introduction by L. A. May, 1977. Oceanside, N.Y.: Dabor Science Publicns.
Ryan, Michael. 1831. *A manual of medical jurisprudence. . . .* London: Renshaw & Rush.
______. 1836. *A manual of medical jurisprudence. . . .* London: Sherwood, Gilbert, & Piper.
Ryan, W. B. 1862. *Infanticide: its law, prevalence, prevention, and history*. London: J. Churchill.
Rymer, Thomas. 1710. *Foedera. . . .* London: A. & J. Churchill.
Sauer, R. 1978. Infanticide and abortion in nineteenth-century Britain. *Popul. Studies*. 32:81–93.
Savitt, T. L. 1979. The social and medical history of crib death. *J. Fla. Med. Assn.* 66:853–59.
Sayles, G. O. 1936. *Select cases in the Court of King's Bench under Edward I*. London: Bernard Quaritch. Selden Soc. 55.
______. 1971. *Select cases in the Court of King's Bench under Richard II, Henry IV and Henry V*. London: Bernard Quaritsch. Selden Soc. 88.
Schreyer, Johann. 1690. *Erörterung und Erläuterung der Frage: Ob es ein gewiss Zeichen, wenn eines todten Kindes Lunge im Wasser untersincket, dass solches in Mutter-Leibe gestorben sey?* Zeitz: J. H. Ammersbach.
Scull, A. T. 1979. *Museums of madness. . . .* New York: St. Martin's.
Severn, Charles. 1831. *First lines of the practice of midwifery. . . .* London: S. Highley.
Simpson, J. Y. 1847a. Discovery of a new anaesthetic agent more efficient than sulphuric ether. *London Med. Gaz.* N.s. 5:934–37.
______. 1847b. On a new anaesthetic agent, more efficient than sulphuric ether. *Lancet*. 2:549–50.
Simpson, Keith. 1961. The development of scientific methods in crime investigation. *J. Forensic Med.* 8:148–56.
______. 1969. The history of scientific crime investigation. *Criminologist*. 4:51–58.
______. 1975. *Forensic medicine*. London: Edward Arnold.
______. 1978. *Forty years of murder*. London: Harrap.
Skae, David. [1840]. *Cases in legal medicine. . . .* Edinburgh: J. Stark.
Smith, F. B. 1979. *The people's health 1830–1900*. New York: Holmes & Meier.
Smith, J. G. 1821. *The principles of forensic medicine. . . .* London: Underwood.
______. 1825. *An analysis of medical evidence. . . .* London: Thomas & George Underwood.
______. 1829. *The claims of forensic medicine. . . .* London: John Taylor.
Smith, Roger. 1981. *Trial by medicine. . . .* Edinburgh: Edinburgh University Press.
Smith, Sydney. 1928. The importance of training in forensic medicine. *J. State Med.* 36:447–61.
______. 1951. The history and development of forensic medicine. *Brit. Med. J.* 1:599–607.
______. 1954. The development of forensic medicine and law-science relations. *J. Public Law* 3:304–18.
Smyth, Frank. 1980. *Cause of death: The story of forensic medicine*. London: Orbis.
Snow, John. 1847. *On the inhalation of the vapour of ether in surgical operations*. London: J. Churchill.
______. 1850. The alleged employment of chloroform by thieves. *London Med. Gaz.* N.s. 10:327.
Spigelius, Adrianus. 1626. *De formato foetu*. Padua: Martini & Pasquato.

1839. Statistics of poisoning in England. *Lancet.* 1:597–99.
1817. *The statutes of the realm.* [N.p.].
1828. *Statutes.* . . . London: H. M. Statute & Law Printers.
1837. *Statutes.* . . . London: H. M. Printers.
Stephen, J. F. 1883. *A history of the criminal law of England.* London: Macmillan.
———. 1890. *A general view of the criminal law of England.* London: Macmillan.
Stow, John. 1970. *Stow's survey of London.* New York: Dutton.
Stuart, Malcolm, ed. 1979. *The encyclopedia of herbs and herbalism.* London: Orbis.
Styles, John. 1983. Sir John Fielding and the problem of criminal investigation in eighteenth-century England. *Trans. Roy. Histor. Soc.* 5th ser. 33:127–49.
1940. A suspected case of leprosy. *Lancet.* 2:441.
Susser, Mervyn, and Abraham Adelstein. 1975. Introduction. In *Vital statistics.* . . . Metuchen, N.J.: Scarecrow Press.
Swammerdamus, Johannis. 1667. *Tractatus physico-anatomico-medicus de respiratione.* . . . Leyden: Gaasbeeck.
Taylor, A. S. 1836. *Elements of medical jurisprudence.* London: Deacon.
———. 1838. Observations and experiments on the lungs of new-born children, in relation to medical jurisprudence. In *Medical and Surgical Monographs.* Philadelphia: A. Waldie.
———. 1844a. *A manual of medical jurisprudence.* London: Churchill.
———. 1844b. Report on the progress of toxicology, in relation to medical jurisprudence, medical police, chemistry, and pharmacy, for the years 1843–44. *Brit. & Foreign Med. Rev.* 18:533–64.
———. 1848. *On poisons in relation to medical jurisprudence and medicine.* London: Churchill.
———. 1856. *Medical jurisprudence.* Philadelphia: Blanchard & Lea.
———. 1860. On the transference of poisons from the blood to the alimentary canal. *Guy's Hosp. Rpts.* 3rd ser. 6:397–403.
———. 1865. *The principles and practice of medical jurisprudence.* London: Churchill.
———. 1869. On homicidal and suicidal wounds of the throat. *Guy's Hosp. Rpts.* Reprinted with Keith Simpson. Some medico-legal comments. Addendum. 1969. *Guy's Hosp. Rpts.* 118:495–515.
———, and G. O. Rees. 1856. The Rugeley suspected secret poisoning cases: Evidence of Dr. Taylor in the case of Ann Palmer, before the coroner's inquest. *Lancet.* 1:78–80, 134–35.
———, and [Samuel] Wilks. 1863. On the cooling of the human body after death: Inferences respecting the time of death. Observations of temperature made in 100 cases. *Guy's Hosp. Rpts.* 3rd ser. 9:180–211.
Taylor, H. L. 1974. The evolution of legal medicine. *Med.-Leg. Bull.* 23:1–7.
Thomas, A. H., ed. 1924. *Calendar of early Mayor's Court rolls . . . a.d. 1298–1307.* Cambridge: Cambridge University Press.
———. 1929. *Calendar of plea and memoranda rolls . . . a.d. 1364–1381.* Cambridge: Cambridge University Press.
———. 1943. *Calendar of plea and memoranda rolls . . . a.d. 1413–1437.* Cambridge: Cambridge University Press.
Thomas, Frederic. 1974. Milestones in forensic science. *J. Forensic Sci.* 19:241–54.
Thomson, A. T. 1831. *Lecture introductory to the course of medical jurisprudence.* . . . London: John Taylor.
———. 1837. Lectures on medical jurisprudence. . . . Lecture XVII. *Lancet.* 1:625–30.
Thorne, S. E., trans. 1968. *Bracton on the laws and customs of England.* Cambridge, Mass.: Belknap.

Thorwald, Jürgen. 1965. *The century of the detective*. New York: Harcourt Brace & World.
Thurston, Gavin. 1969. A queer sort of thing. *Med.-Leg. J.* 37:165–71.
Traill, T. S. 1836. *Outlines of a course of lectures on medical jurisprudence*. Edinburgh: Black.
1829. Trial of Mr. Van Butchell for manslaughter. *London Med. Gaz.* 4:89–93.
Tuke, D. H. 1909. Prichard, James Cowles. In Sidney Lee, ed. *Dictionary of national biography*. New York: Macmillan.
1659. *The unhappy marksman*. London: T. N. for R. Clavell. Reprinted 1809. Harleian Miscell. 4:1–12.
1860. Unwholesome meat. *Lancet*. 2:448.
Valentini, M. B. 1722. *Corpus juris medico-legale*. Frankfurt am Main: J. A. Jung.
Virchow, R. L. K. 1858. *Die Cellularpathologie*. . . . Berlin: A. Hirschwald.
1875a. The Wainwright case in its medico-legal aspects. *Brit. Med. J.* 2:735–37.
1875b. The Wainwright case: Dr. Meadows on the post mortem diagnosis of a multiparous uterus. *Brit. Med. J.* 2:744.
Waldo, F. J. 1904. Notes on some remarkable British cases of criminal poisoning. *Med. Brief.* 32:175–82, 253–59, 452–58, 936–40.
Walker, Nigel. 1968. *Crime and insanity in England. Vol. 1, The historical perspective*. Edinburgh: Edinburgh University Press.
———, and Sarah McCabe. [1968]. *Crime and insanity in England. Volume 2, New solutions and new problems*. Edinburgh: Edinburgh University Press.
Wallis, J. E. P., ed. 1892. Trial of Daniel M'Naghten. *Reports of state trials*. N. s. 4:847–48, 926–34. London: Eyre & Spottiswoode.
Walsh, J. J. 1819. *History of medicine in New York*. New York, National Americana Soc.
Watkins, John. 1815. *Important results of an elaborate investigation into the mysterious case of Elizabeth Fenning*. . . . London: W. Hone.
Watson, Alexander. 1842. *Medico-legal treatise on homicide by external violence*. . . . Edinburgh: Maclachlan, Stewart.
Waugh, M. A. 1973. Venereal diseases in sixteenth-century England. *Med. Hist.* 17:192–99.
Webster, James. 1824. *An essay on medical jurisprudence*. Philadelphia: Wm. Brown.
Welsch, Gottfried. 1660. *Rationale vulnerum lethalium judicium*. Leipzig: Ritzsch.
Wepfer, J. J. 1658. *Observationes anatomicae, ex cadaveribus eorum, quos sustulit apoplexia*. . . . Schaffhausen: J. C. Suter.
Wharton, Francis, and Moreton Stillé. 1855. *A treatise on medical jurisprudence*. Rochester, N.Y.: Lawyer's Co-operative.
Wheatley, H. B., and Peter Cunningham. 1891. *London past and present*. . . . London: John Murray.
White, Beatrice. 1965. *Cast of ravens*. . . . New York: George Braziller.
Wiecking, D. K. 1979. The legal importance of a dying declaration. *Med.-Leg. Bull.* 28:1–5.
Willcock, J. H. 1830. *The laws relating to the medical profession*. . . . London: A. Strahan.
Williams, S. W. 1835. *A catechism of medical jurisprudence*. . . . Northampton, Mass.: J. H. Butler.
Willis, Thomas. 1664. *Cerebri anatome*. . . . London: J. Flesher.
Willis, Thomas, trans. 1847. *The works of William Harvey*. London: Sydenham Soc.
Winslow, Forbes. 1843. *The plea of insanity in criminal cases*. London: H. Renshaw.
Woodman, W. B., and C. M. Tidy. 1877. *Forensic medicine and toxicology*. Philadelphia: Lindsay & Blakiston.

Wormley, T. G. 1867. *Micro-chemistry of poisons. . . .* New York: Baillière.
Wrightson, Keith. 1975. Infanticide in earlier seventeenth-century England. *Popul. Stud.* No. 15:10–22.
Wunderli, Richard. 1982. Pre-Reformation London summoners and the murder of Richard Hunne. *J. Eccles. History.* 33:209–24.
Young, J. H. 1979. "Even to a sucking infant": Nostrums and children. *Trans. Stud. Coll. Physicians Phila.* 5th ser. 1:5–32.
Zacchia, Paolo. 1621–35, 1666. *Quaestiones medico-legales. . . .* 1621–35, Rome: G. Facciotti; 1666, Amsterdam: J. Blaev.
Zittman, J. F. 1706. *Medicina forensis.* Frankfurt am Main: Sumptibus Societatis.

Index

Index